CALIFORNIA STATE UNIVERSITY, SACRAMENTO

This book is due on the last date stamped below.
Failure to return books on the date due will result in assessment
of overdue fees.

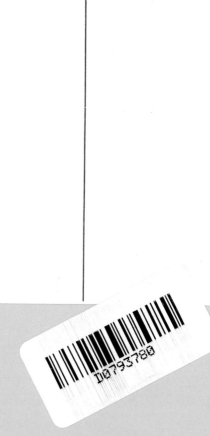

Psychopharmacology of Cognitive and Psychiatric Disorders in the Elderly

Psychopharmacology of Cognitive and Psychiatric Disorders in the Elderly

Edited by

David Wheatley

Stamford Psychiatric Clinic
(formerly Royal Masonic Hospital)
Ravenscourt Park. London
W6 0TN

and

David Smith

Texas A&M University
Health Science Center
College of Medicine
Temple Campus
Brownwood
Texas 76801
USA

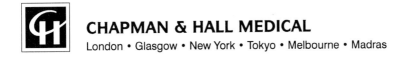

CHAPMAN & HALL MEDICAL
London • Glasgow • New York • Tokyo • Melbourne • Madras

Published by Chapman & Hall, 2–6 Boundary Row, London SE1 8HN, UK

Chapman & Hall, 2–6 Boundary Row, London SE1 8HN, UK

Chapman & Hall GmbH, Pappelallee 3, 69469 Weinheim, Germany

Chapman & Hall USA, 115 Fifth Avenue, New York, NY 10003, USA

Chapman & Hall Japan, ITP-Japan, Kyowa Building, 3F, 2-2-1 Hirakawacho, Chiyoda-ku, Tokyo 102, Japan

Chapman & Hall Australia, 102 Dodds Street, South Melbourne, Victoria 3205, Australia

Chapman & Hall India, R. Seshadri, 32 Second Main Road, CIT East, Madras 600 035, India

First edition 1998

© 1998

Typeset in 10/12pt Palatino by Saxon Graphics Ltd

Printed in Great Britain by St Edmundsbury Press, Bury St Edmunds

ISBN 0 412 82470 1

A catalogue record for this book is available from the British Library

Library of Congress Catalog Card Number: 97-69680

∞ Printed on permanent acid-free text paper, manufactured in accordance with ANSI/NISO Z39.48-1992 and ANSI/NISO Z39.48-1984 (Permanence of Paper).

Contents

Contributors

Robin A. Braithwaite
Regional Laboratory for Toxicology
City Hospital NHS Teaching Trust
Dudley Road
Birmingham
B18 7QH, UK

Davis Coakley
Robert Mayne Day Hospital
St James's Hospital
Dublin 8
Eire

Albert Enz
Novartis Pharma
CH-400 Basel
Switzerland

Danielle Fallin
Roskamp Laboratory
Department of Psychiatry and Behavioral Medicine
University of Southern Florida
3515 E Fletcher Ave, Tampa
Florida 33613

Julian Gray
Praecis Pharmaceuticals
1 Hampshire Street, 5th Floor
Cambridge
MA 02139
USA

Robin Holliday
CSIRO Molecular Science
Sydney Laboratory
P.O. Box 184
North Ryde
Sydney, NSW 2113
Australia

Antony Hordern
5 Banks Avenue
North Turramurra
New South Wales
Sydney, Australia
NSW, 2074

Anita Kotak
Imperial College School of Medicine at St Mary's Hospital
Department of Pharmacology
Norfolk Place
London
W2 1PG, UK

Chris Krasucki
Institute of Psychiatry
De Crespigny Park
Denmark Hill
London
SE5 8AF, UK

Malcolm H. Lader
Institute of Psychiatry
De Crespigny Park
London
SE5 8AF, UK

Stuart A. Montgomery
Imperial College School of Medicine at St Mary's Hospital
Department of Pharmacology
Norfolk Place
London
W2 1PG, UK

Declan McLoughlin
Institute of Psychiatry
De Crespigny Park
Denmark Hill
London, SE5 8AF

Michael Mullan
Roskamp Laboratory
Department of Psychiatry and Behavioral Medicine
University of Southern Florida
3515 E Fletcher Avenue, Tampa
Florida 33613

Denis O'Mahony
Department of Geriatric Medicine
University of Birmingham
Selly Oak Hospital
Raddlebarn Road
Birmingham
B29 6JD, UK

M.S. John Pathy
Healthcare Research Unit
St Wodos Hospital
Newport
Gwent
NP9 4SZ, UK

Brice Pitt
Department of Psychological Medicine
Hammersmith Hospital
Du Cane Road
London
W12 0HA, UK

Lon S. Schneider
Department of Psychiatry and Behavioral Sciences
Geriatric Studies Clinic
1975 Zonal Avenue, KAM-400
Los Angeles
CA 90033
USA

David A. Smith
Texas A & M University
Health Science Center
College of Medicine
Temple Campus
Brownwood
Texas 76801
USA

Pierre N. Tariot
University of Rochester Medical Center
Department of Psychiatry
435 E. Henrietta Road
Rochester
NY 14620
USA

Nancy Tresser
Roskamp Laboratory
Department of Psychiatry and Behavioral Medicine
University of Southern Florida
3515 E Fletcher Avenue, Tampa
Florida 33613

David Wheatley
Stamford Psychiatric Clinic
(formerly Royal Masonic Hospital), Ravenscourt Park
London
W6 0TN, UK

Foreword

Since 'The Psychopharmacology of Old Age' was published in 1982 the population of the world has continued to grow and, with the decline in mortality from cardiovascular diseases in particular, an increasing number of people are reaching advanced age. The rate of population growth peaked in the late 1960s at just over 2% per annum. In 1997 the world has approximately 5.7 billion people. The next century is expected to end with about 11 billion people, after which population growth may become stationary. It is estimated that approximately one-fifth of the world's population is now living in extreme poverty, i.e. living with a level of income or expenditure below which a minimum, nutritionally adequate diet and essential non-food requirements cannot be obtained. This situation is commonest in the poor countries of the developing world. Extreme poverty is associated with poor health, a reduced lifestyle and premature mortality.

Between 1945 and 1995 the global expectation of life increased from 43 to 66 years. These gains, greatest in the developed world, were due to public health measures, higher material living standards, education and biomedical advances. The expectation of life for females and for males in Australia is now 81 and 75 years, respectively; in the United Kingdom it is 79 and 74 years; in the United States it is 79 and 72 years. The Japanese, however, live the longest: female expectation of life is 83 years and males can expect to reach the age of 76 years. The goals of geriatric medicine are the prevention of functional decline on the one hand and the preservation of functional independence on the other. With improvements in the health of elderly people, due to their healthier lifestyles with better diets, adequate exercise, avoidance of smoking and the treatment of readily managed disorders such as hypertension, hyperlipidaemia and, in many cases, coronary artery disease, it has become possible to talk of the 'young old' and the 'old old' who present different problems for the medical profession.

In countries of the developed world particularly, older members of the population tend to be disadvantaged in that much of their expertise is

constantly being made obsolete by advances in technology. In our tech-
nosociety the virtues of youth, energy and physical beauty are lauded to
the detriment of the older, more solid, virtues such as conscientiousness,
reliability and benevolence. In daily living the old frequently experience
difficulty in coping with electronic devices such as the programming of
VCRs and the operation of computers. These skills are rapidly acquired
by the young who find it hard to understand the difficulties their elders
have encountered. Many young people who have grown up in today's
world are self-centred and see no reason why, through taxes and charita-
ble institutions, they should support the care of those elderly who are in
need of assistance and medical treatment. This is likely to become an
increasing problem as populations age and the reducing proportion of
those who are working have to meet the expense of caring for the more
numerous elderly.

Psychiatric illness is common in old age and often presents in combination with physical disease(s) and social problems. 'Losses' which contribute
to psychiatric disorders increase with age whether they are physical, such
as losses of strength and dexterity, reduction in mobility, impairment of
vision, auditory problems or psychological ones such as the deaths of dear
ones, retirement, reduced financial circumstances, loneliness and so forth.
The authors of the chapters in 'Psychopharmacology of Cognitive and
Psychiatric Disorders in the Elderly' have critically surveyed this vast field
which is destined to become even more vast in the foreseeable future, bar-
ring some enormous natural disaster or some man-made horror such as
nuclear or biological warfare. The nature of ageing is reviewed, as are the
pharmacokinetics of drug treatment of the elderly and the adverse effects
that such drugs can produce. For obvious reasons much interest has
focused in recent years on the dementias, particularly Alzheimer's disease.
Although effective treatment for this common disorder is not available,
knowledge is accruing of likely risk factors and of possible protective and
delaying strategies such as, in women, the administration of oestrogen during and after the menopause. Depression is particularly important in old
age because it is common and widespread, is often missed or misdiagnosed
as dementia and because a variety of effective safe antidepressant drugs
are now available to treat it. The advent of these drugs from the late 1950s
onwards, together with the availability of the tranquillizers and lithium,
has given great impetus to geriatric psychopharmacology and has con-
tributed significantly to ameliorating the lot of many old people burdened
with mental illnesses.

Anthony Hordern
North Turramurra, NSW, Australia

Part One

Basic Concepts

1

The causes of ageing

Robin Holliday

INTRODUCTION

It is widely believed that ageing is a major unsolved problem in biology. I argue here that this is mistaken, and that a broad view which encompasses a considerable proportion of the whole of biological knowledge makes it clear why ageing exists in mammals and many other animals. There are three basic questions. Why do we age? Why do we live as long as we do? Why do different mammalian species have very different maximum lifespans? In answering these questions, a great deal is revealed about the mechanisms which underpin eventual senescence and death. Almost all the material in this chapter will be found in *Understanding Ageing* [1], which is fully referenced. For the most part, these references are omitted here.

Origins of biological ageing

The evolution of multicellular organisms, or metazoans, leads to the differentiation of cells that perform specific functions. Some of these cells become post-mitotic, that is, they lose the ability to divide further. In early animals it is likely that there was a pool of totipotent cells, which could divide and differentiate and which could replace differentiated cells, should these become damaged or killed. Simple animals that exist today, such as coelenterates and flatworms, have this property. These animals do not age, at least in the usual sense, because they have the ability to regenerate all parts of the organism. Sexual reproduction also exists in most of these species, so we see, side by side, the transmission of germ line cells from generation to generation, and also a pool of totipotent

Psychopharmacology of Cognitive and Psychiatric Disorders in the Elderly. Edited by David Wheatley and David Smith. Published in 1998 by Chapman and Hall, London. ISBN 0 412 82470 1

somatic cells which can maintain the body for a very long period or indefinitely. A large number of present day plants also have these regenerative abilities.

Darwin realised that most organisms produce more offspring than can possibly survive. Following the lead of Malthus, who made it clear that a continual logarithmic increase in the number of individuals could never be sustained indefinitely, Darwin came to understand that the environment imposes severe limits on reproductive potential. In a hostile ecosystem the fittest organisms are more likely to survive than the less fit. This is the fundamental feature of natural selection. It follows that, of all offspring, only a proportion reach adulthood and amongst these there is a given probability, per unit of time, of death from predation, disease, starvation and drought. An examination of many populations of animals shows that they are *age-structured*, in that cohorts of individuals of increasing age progressively diminish.

We now consider two types of animals, A and B, which are in every way similar except that A does not age, whereas B does. At first sight it would seem that A is fitter in Darwinian terms than B, because adults can reproduce continuously, whereas B can only reproduce for a finite period of time. In a protected environment this may be so, but the reality is that animals live in hostile environments and their survival is limited for that reason. What is the specific property that allows A to survive indefinitely in a good environment? It is the ability to *maintain* the soma, or body, by the repair and replacement of damaged or lost cells, tissues or organs. This ability requires considerable investment of metabolic resources. In contrast, animal B is unable to maintain the soma; in other words it has dispensed with some or all of the regenerative resources of animal A. As survival is not prolonged in a real ecosystem, it follows that the resources saved by animal B can instead be invested in reproduction; it is simply a better strategy for survival to develop to an adult, reproduce during the limited time available and not attempt to maintain the soma indefinitely.

This happened during animal evolution. Indeed, in many animals, such as insects and nematodes (roundworms), an adult body has evolved where *all* the somatic cells are post-mitotic and cannot be replaced. As we see later, non-dividing cells cannot be expected to survive indefinitely. A body architecture in which all cells are post-mitotic leads to a clearly defined limit to survival, and ageing is particularly well-defined in organisms such as insects and nematodes. We can therefore conclude that ageing is of ancient origin, and probably evolved concomitantly with the emergence of many invertebrate animals. In the animal kingdom as a whole, there is enormous diversity in lifestyle as well as in the longevities of adults. This chapter focuses on the ageing of humans and other mammalian species.

BRIEF HISTORY OF RESEARCH ON AGEING

In the last century, August Weismann published the earliest scientific discussions on animal ageing. He realised that germ line cells are potentially immortal cells whereas the cells of the soma are finite. The distinction between germ line and soma is accepted as a key feature of animal biology, but the distinction is much less clear in plants. Weismann also discussed the evolution of ageing, but Medawar [2] and others have explained that his views were largely erroneous. Weismann's contributions released a flood of speculation about the nature and causes of ageing. Comfort [3] briefly surveyed this work and concludes that little of it has any substance. Serious experimental studies of ageing began in this century and have continued with a variety of animal systems, including protozoa, flatworms, rotifers, nematodes, insects (especially *Drosophila*), fish and mammals. This work has been reviewed by Comfort [4] and more recently by Finch [5].

Experimental studies fall into two broad categories. On the one hand investigators have made comparisons between young and old animals. They have examined many morphological, physiological or biochemical parameters using cells, tissues, organs or whole animals. Large differences between young and old animals have been documented. The reasons for these differences are not clear; indeed, many of the observations made cannot be interpreted. On the other hand, scientists have tried to test particular theories of ageing, with the parameter investigated expected to change in the direction predicted by the theory. The results have rarely been clear cut, probably because no single theory explains ageing. More recently, considerable attention has been paid to the ageing of human cells in culture. Again, an enormous amount of information is available, but the elucidation of the actual causes of the ageing of these cells remains elusive. In my view, some of the most rewarding experimental studies of mammalian ageing have been comparative, that is, the investigation of a particular parameter in a range of related species with very different lifespans. In many cases these have provided evidence that longevity is related to the efficiency of maintenance of the organism. The results are reviewed later.

The accepted gerontological literature excludes the vast range of studies on the pathological changes often seen in aged people. This is an anomaly because so much information has been published about human cells, tissues and organs, throughout the human lifespan. It is evident to everyone that many serious pathological conditions are age-related or age-associated, yet both the gerontologists and the clinicians have separated this extensive documentation in humans from the study of ageing itself. This stems from the erroneous view that 'natural ageing' is in some way distinct from disease. As biological ageing cannot itself be regarded as 'a disease', it has also been assumed that the diseases of old age have little to do with ageing itself. The time has come to establish the relationship of ageing to the diseases which occur predominantly in later life. This will demand a different attitude, particularly amongst biomedical scientists. The aetiology of age-related disease will only be understood by more basic research on ageing itself [6].

THE EVOLVED DESIGN OF MAMMALIAN ORGANISMS

Amongst the cold-blooded vertebrates (fish, amphibia and reptiles) there is an enormous diversity in lifestyles and lifespans. Some small fish live about one year, whereas others survive many decades. The latter keep growing throughout their lifespan, as do some of the largest reptiles, such as tortoises and crocodiles. Although this continual growth is associated with long lifespans, these are, of course, only a minute fraction of evolutionary time. With the evolution of warmblooded (or homothermic) mammals and birds, a more uniform pattern of ageing became prevalent. Growth is normally completed in young adults capable of reproduction. After a period of normal fertility, reproduction slows down or ceases, and this is followed by the gradual onset of senescence and death. In both mammals and birds, there is an approximately 50-fold difference between the shortest and longest lived species, but the three stages of life: growth, reproduction and senescence, are common throughout.

The vast amount of information we have about the cells, tissues and organs of mammalian and to a lesser extent avian species, explains why survival of the adult is fairly well defined. The adult brain consists of non-dividing neurons, with a number of cells, such as glial cells or astrocytes, capable of division. Brain function depends on these neurons, which cannot divide. They are in quasi-steady state, that is, they can retain normal function for long periods but, with time, the steady state is gradually lost. Damage may occur in the chromosomal DNA, abnormal proteins are not always removed and mitochondria lose normal function. The number of normal neurons gradually declines throughout the lifespan, so the brain necessarily has a limit to survival. The heart is a very efficient pump, but like the brain it has a poor ability to renew and repair itself. The myotubes are post-mitotic muscle cells that are not replaceable. Similarly, the anatomy of the major blood vessels is not conducive to successful and ongoing repair. The analogy with a machine is apt in this context. It can be designed to last a long time, but eventually breakdown is inevitable. Before this happens, however, the machine may be shut down, repaired and restarted for another long period. This is not possible, of course, in the case of the heart and vascular system which is designed to 'last a lifetime' only.

Many proteins in the mammalian body are extremely long-lived. The crystallins of the lens are laid down early in life and are never replaced. Many abnormal modifications can occur in protein molecules, including oxidation, cross-linking, non-enzymic glycosylation, racemisation of individual amino acids, deamidation and partial denaturation. These occur in lens proteins and may eventually lead to cataract formation. Similarly, collagen molecules, the various forms of which comprise the commonest protein in the body, are very long-lived. Yet these molecules turn over very slowly and many become progressively cross-linked with age. This cross-linking has been much studied and is one of the best biomarkers of ageing. Since the molecules are rarely replaced, the progressive changes in collagen have serious effects on the body tissues and organs such as loss of skin elasticity, increased friction and wear in joints, and slower wound healing. Together with similar changes in another long-lived protein, elastin, cross-linking leads to hardening of the arteries, an increase in blood pressure and all the consequences that can arise from these changes.

There are other body components that can be expected to last a lifetime but not forever, and the teeth are a very good example. These are 'programmed' by our genes to be of sufficient size and strength, but nevertheless they are subject to wear and tear throughout life, and eventually they are worn down or lost. Milk teeth are replaced by adult teeth and, in principle, there is no biological reason why a lost adult tooth should not be replaced by a new one; but we did not evolve that way, instead we are dependant on dentists for ongoing tooth function. Similarly the retina of the eye is not capable of repair and replacement. The photoreceptors in the post-mitotic rods and cones continually turn over during one's lifetime. Much of the protein is degraded and removed by the underlying layer of epithelial cells, but this is not a steady-state system and eventually insoluble proteins and lipofuscin accumulate in these cells. Retinopathy is a common condition in old age.

A remarkable feature of ageing is the decline in organ and tissue function that occurs with a broad degree of synchrony. There is no direct connection between collagen cross-linking, loss of neurons or the wearing down of teeth, but all occur at the same time together with many other deleterious changes in the body. It is reasonable to conclude that there are multiple causes of ageing, but there is an overall control determined by many genes.

MAINTENANCE OF THE ORGANISM

Of the three fairly well-defined periods in the total lifespan, the first two, development and reproduction, are crucial for survival of the species. The adult is maintained in a normal physiological state during the period of reproduction, and the effectiveness of this maintenance will determine the final lifespan. There are at least 10 major maintenance mechanisms, which together comprise a very significant proportion of all metabolic resources.

DNA repair

Although DNA is a stable molecule, it is prone to so-called 'spontaneous' damage and also to damage from extrinsic agents such as UV light or chemicals in the food. To maintain the functional integrity of cells, the structure of DNA is preserved by an elaborate system of repair enzymes. These were first discovered in micro-organisms such as *Escherichia coli*, but enough is now known to be sure that a comparable set of enzymes exist in mammalian cells. It is clear that considerable resources are used to detect defects in DNA, to remove the abnormality and to fill in the gap with normal DNA bases. One of the commonest lesions in DNA is the apurinic gap (the loss of a purine residue), and it has been estimated that there may be 10 000 of these per cell per day, most of which are effectively repaired. It has been suggested that those chemical lesions that are relatively uncommon are not repaired and may continually accumulate, especially in non-dividing cells [7].

The synthesis of macromolecules

It is well known that DNA synthesis is extremely accurate, with only one error per 10^8 to 10^{10} base pairs. Thus, on average, each cell division may generate about one error or mutation in the whole human genome (6×10^9 base pairs). This is achieved by proof-reading or editing processes, whereby initial errors in replication are recognised and eliminated. In this regard, there is some overlap between DNA repair and proof-reading. It is obvious that organisms invest considerable metabolic resources to protect the integrity of their genetic material, but there must be some optimum level of accuracy. It is possible that this optimum is not the same for different species, but we have no information on this point.

The accuracy of RNA and protein synthesis is several orders of magnitude less than that of DNA synthesis. Again, there are proof-reading mechanisms to ensure that resources are not wasted in the synthesis of non-functional molecules. Also, it is essential to avoid a possible instability in translation due to the feedback of errors or defects into the machinery for protein synthesis itself (see below).

Protein turnover

Proteins are subject to a large number of post-synthetic modifications, some of which are normal, but others are abnormal. These latter modifications include oxidation, glycation, cross-linking, deamidation and partial denaturation. There are screening mechanisms which can recognise abnormalities in protein molecules and these trigger proteolytic degradation. This is an ongoing process to ensure that the cell contains mainly normal molecules. As is well known from ageing studies, the accumulation of defective or denatured proteins can have devastating effects on cellular function. The continual turnover of proteins in the body requires considerable metabolic resources and also requires the continual intake of nitrogen (in the form of amino acids) to replace those lost during degradation of proteins which are converted to urea and excreted.

Defences against oxygen free radicals

Respiration and other metabolic processes generate short-lived oxygen free radicals that are highly reactive. These can damage membranes, proteins and DNA. There are two basic defence mechanisms against free radical attack. First, there are enzymes such as superoxide dismutase, catalase, glutathione peroxidase and reductase, which act to remove free radicals. Second, there are antioxidants, or sinks for free radicals. These include ascorbic acid (vitamin C), α-tocopherol (vitamin E), cysteine and glutathione, uric acid, bilirubin, ubiquinol and carnosine. The protein transferrin has an important role in removing free iron, which can efficiently generate dangerous hydroxyl radicals. Carotene is a normal component of diet and it is an active sink for free radicals.

The suggestion that damage from oxygen free radicals may be an important component of ageing was made over 40 years ago, but only recently has the theory become very fashionable. There is new extensive research on the generation of free radicals, the damage they produce and the defences against this damage. There is also much interest in the damage suffered by the mitochondrial genome, which is a particularly sensitive target, as oxygen free radicals are a by-product of the respiratory activity of mitochondria.

Toxic chemicals and detoxification

A natural diet contains not only required nutrients but also a variety of chemicals which can be harmful to the body. These typically come from plants, which produce a very wide range of toxic compounds to protect themselves from animals. The major defence mechanism is a large family of mono-oxygenase enzymes known as the p450 cytochromes. These carry out a multiplicity of chemical reactions, which collectively remove toxic chemicals in the diet. The liver is the major site of detoxification but it also occurs in other locations. In many cases, the necessary enzyme is induced by the toxic chemical that is subsequently destroyed. In the detoxification process, active intermediates are often produced which are rapidly converted to inactive compounds and excreted. Much research in the field stems from the fact that active intermediates (including those from man-made chemicals) can be potent carcinogens. For example, hydrocarbons can be converted to oxidised forms which damage DNA. Clearly the p450 cytochromes have evolved to deal with normal toxins, and they may be less efficient at removing the many man-made chemicals in our environment.

The immune response

Immunology is a science in its own right and it is taken for granted that it is one of our major defence and maintenance mechanisms. Large slow feeding animals are continually subject to attack by rapidly reproducing pathogenic viruses, bacteria and animal parasites. There has been strong selection for a whole battery of cellular and chemical defence mechanisms which together constitute the immune system. A striking feature of this response is that there are several lines of defence so that if one fails there is commonly a backup mechanism. The importance of the immune system for the normal maintenance of the adult body is shown by patients who develop the symptoms of AIDS. In this case the eventual destruction of CD4 lymphocytes allows the pathogen to overwhelm the patient.

Wound healing

Lower vertebrates have considerable powers of regeneration. For example, some amphibian species can regenerate an amputated leg. In mammals, dramatic regeneration of this type has been lost, but very significant wound healing ability remains. Light skin damage is repaired all the time and leaves no scars. More severe damage also results in effective repair but with the formation of scar tissue. Prior to the healing process the blood clotting mechanism comes into play. This is important, especially in haemophiliacs, to prevent bleeding from open wounds as well as internal ones. Tissues vary greatly in their capacity to repair damage. The brain and central nervous system have a very limited capacity, as do the heart and major blood vessels. In contrast, skeletal muscle can regenerate from the pool of myoblasts differentiating into myotubes, and broken bones can be repaired. During evolution, a balance has been struck between the investment of resources into important ongoing repair of damage from various hazards and a reduction or loss of the ability to replace limbs and major organs.

Epigenetic controls

Much less is known about this maintenance mechanism, but it is of fundamental importance. When the embryo develops, cells differentiate into specialised types, with or without the ability to divide further. These specialised cells have a very stable phenotype which is dependent on the activity of a given set of genes, producing proteins characteristic of that cell type. Once a cell is fully differentiated it remains in that state. Some of these cells are able to divide (e.g. fibroblasts, lymphocytes), whereas others never do so (neurons, myotubes). The mechanisms which turn on one set of genes specific for one cell types and turn off those genes specific for all other cell type are not well understood. One likely mechanism depends on the methylation of cytosine in DNA, as it has been shown in many contexts that silent genes have methylated promoter sequences. Such mechanisms, which do not depend on changes in DNA sequence, are referred to as *epigenetic*. It is obvious that maintenance of the integrity of body cells and tissues depends on the efficient control of gene activities. It is also obvious that loss of such controls can have disastrous consequences, in particular the development of tumours. Such cells have lost some of their normal regulatory controls and become to a lesser or greater extent de-differentiated. Genes have been identified which play important roles in the maintenance of normal cell phenotypes. Mutations in such genes, when inherited, predispose the individual to a higher incidence of cancer.

Apoptosis

It is now well recognised that a special mechanism exists to remove unwanted cells. This self-destruct mechanism, apoptosis, is triggered in a variety of contexts. Apoptosis occurs during normal development, for example during the morphogenesis of the digits of the hand and foot. It is also a normal part of the emergence of the central nervous and immune systems, during which unwanted cells are discarded. However, it is also a maintenance system in the sense that cells which are damaged or abnormal often switch on the apoptotic process. Otherwise such cells would survive and might harm the organism. Although it has sometimes been suggested that apoptosis and ageing are linked, there is little if any evidence for increased apoptosis during ageing. It may well be that the reverse is true, that is, abnormal cells which are normally killed off by apoptosis may survive during ageing. If this were correct, it would imply that the efficiency of the switching mechanism or apoptosis itself may decline with age.

Homeostatic mechanisms

Homeostatis comprises a very large number of physiological or regulatory processes that maintain the body in a normal functional state. The most important homeostatic mechanism in mammals and birds is a constant body temperature, which produces a more uniform environment than occurs in cold-blooded vertebrates. The body is more independent of the environment and can therefore function normally over a range of external temperatures. Moreover, a uniform internal temperature allows the evolution of optimised physiological systems, with many proteins closely adapted to that temperature. The control of temperature is itself a maintenance mechanism, but there are also innumerable other homeostatic controls. Some are based on hormones, such as insulin which is essential for the control of blood sugar levels. Others may be triggered by the animals' activity, for example increased oxygen uptake following the increased use of muscles. Some are based on cellular responses. The loss of blood results in an increased production of blood cells, and low oxygen content at high altitudes leads to an increased production of erythrocytes. Responses to environmental stress may be rapid. For example, exposure to high temperature results in the synthesis of 'heat shock proteins', which protect cells from the effects of heat. Also, DNA damage induces the p53 protein, the so-called 'guardian of the genome', which blocks the cell cycle until the damage is repaired.

Physiological homeostasis is essential for the maintenance of normal body function, and cellular homeostasis comprises the battery of regulatory mechanisms which allow individual cells to perform normally and also allow them to interact with other cells. The multiple ways that cells interact and influence each other is a major area of current research. If maintenance mechanisms are essential for the preservation of homeostasis and normal survival, then ultimately they determine the length of life: the more efficient they are, the longer an animal will live. It follows from this that failure of maintenance and loss of homeostasis may result in death. As there are multiple maintenance mechanisms, it follows that there are multiple causes of ageing.

The study of all maintenance mechanisms comprises a major part of biology, yet most such studies are not regarded as being any part of gerontology. Nevertheless, I believe that a full understanding of ageing depends on a knowledge of maintenance and particularly its eventual failure. It is also important to stress that innumerable genes are required for the enzymes and proteins on which maintenance depends. Thus, many many genes influence the lifespan, not just a few as some believe.

THEORIES OF AGEING

It is striking that various theories of ageing relate, in one way or another, to the failure of the major maintenance mechanisms that have been outlined. For example, the somatic mutation theory relates to DNA repair mechanisms and in particular the failure of repair or error-prone repair. The free radical theory of ageing relates to the failure of the defences against oxygen free radicals. In consequence, damage to DNA, proteins and membranes occurs. The protein error theory proposes that mistakes in protein synthesis may feed back into transcription and translation, thus causing further errors. Accuracy in macromolecule synthesis is a defence against this happening. There is no doubt that abnormal proteins accumulate in a variety of contexts during ageing, and there are theories that propose that the failure to remove such proteins is a major cause of ageing. The 'dysdifferentiation' theory is based on the supposition that epigenetic controls are relaxed during ageing and this gives rise to the synthesis of 'ectopic proteins', which can have deleterious effects. The efficiency of the immune system declines during ageing, and the 'immunologic' theory of ageing proposes that a progressive failure to distinguish self from non-self antigens leads to a variety of autoimmune responses, some of which have pathological effects. It was suggested long ago that toxic chemicals in the gut may be an important cause of senescence; there are many who believe today that diet may have a strong influences on longevity. If this were so, then the efficiency of detoxification is a key player in determining lifespan. Finally, there are neuroendocrine theories of ageing which propose that major homeostatic mechanisms change during ageing, and these can be linked to programmed ageing or the concept of a pacemaker or clock that determines the lifespan (see below).

As these theories of ageing relate quite closely to failure of various maintenance mechanisms, all of which are essential for survival, I believe that there is likely to be some truth in all the theories mentioned. A more global view, which encompasses all or several theories, is far preferable to the narrow view which protagonists of individual theories tend to adopt. This may explain the failure of most attempts to test specific theories of ageing. It could be argued that some theories provide 'primary' explanations (e.g. somatic mutations, protein errors), whereas others are secondary (e.g. the decline of the immune system). Why does the immune system decline with age? Of all cell and organ systems it seems to have the greatest potential for renewal. So one needs to suppose that key cells have limited lifespan, in terms of either their chronological survival or their proliferative potential. What then determines their lifespan?

A better approach is to propose that failure of maintenance affects cells, which affect tissues, which in turn affect organs. Accumulated changes at the molecular level, whether in DNA, proteins, membranes or organelles, ultimately lead to the disruption of higher order maintenance mechanisms, such as the immune system or physiological homeostasis. An example of this, not yet established, might be the accumulation of defective insulin receptors or the loss of such receptors with age, which in turn lead to late-onset diabetes and all the side-effects that follow.

A distinction is often made between so-called 'programme' theories of ageing and stochastic 'wear and tear' theories. I believe this distinction is unreal, as a few examples will show. The size and strength of teeth is genetically programmed, yet continual use wears them down. The chemistry of collagen and its cross-linking is the same or very similar in humans and rats, yet it occurs much more rapidly in the rat. Presumably the internal milieu of the rat, perhaps related to metabolic rate and the production of oxygen free radicals, favours the formation of cross-links. Similar considerations apply to the lifetime of neurons in the brain, changes in lens crystallins and so on. Almost any parameter we care to look at which changes with age is likely to be the consequence of the genes which determine a particular body component and the maintenance mechanisms, which preserve it or fail to preserve it over a given time scale.

LONGEVITY AND THE FAILURE OF MAINTENANCE

The foregoing discussion leads directly to the prediction that the efficiency of maintenance is related to longevity. A number of comparative studies in different mammalian species strongly support this prediction [1].

1. Somatic cells in culture have finite proliferative potential before senescence sets in. Fibroblasts are the most widely studied cell type and it has been convincingly shown, with these cells from eight mammalian species with very different longevities (from mouse to human), that their *in vitro* lifespan is correlated with the donor organism's lifespan. It is true that we do not fully understand the mechanisms of senescence of these cells, but it is very reasonable to suppose that long-lived species depend on a greater capacity of fibroblasts to survive and multiply *in vivo*. In this connection, it is known that the *in vitro* proliferative potential of fibroblasts from humans or hamsters is *inversely* correlated with donor age.

2. Five comparative studies have been published on the efficiency of repair of DNA damaged by UV light. In four of these the efficiency of repair directly correlated with the lifespans of the mammalian species studied, although one study was ambiguous. (These studies have been critically reviewed by Tice and Setlow [8]). Lens epithelium is exposed to sunlight in a normal environment, so it is satisfying to find (in one of the four positive studies) that these cells from long-lived mammals repair this damage much more effectively than those from short-lived species.

3. Poly ADP ribose polymerase is a ubiquitous enzyme which plays a role in DNA metabolism and repair, although its exact functions remain to be defined. A study of 13 mammalian species showed that enzyme activity is correlated with lifespan. The activity of another enzyme important in DNA metabolism, γ-ray-induced ADP ribosyl transferase, is also correlated with the longevity of mammalian species.

4. Dimethyl benzanthracene (DMBA) is a carcinogen which in its activated form can bind to DNA (see detoxification above). It was found that the extent of binding in fibroblasts is negatively correlated with donor lifespan. This is expected if long-lived species better protect their DNA from intermediates of detoxification, or ensure that such intermediates are destroyed more quickly. In a related study, the mutagenicity of activated DMBA was shown to be inversely correlated with the lifespan of the species.

5. A number of comparative studies have been carried out on oxygen free radical damage or the defences against such damage. These include the measurement of oxidised DNA bases in urine, the concentration of carotenoids in serum, antioxidation and peroxide formation and the activity of superoxide dismutase. In general, these support the prediction that long-lived mammalian species have better defences against free radical damage than short-lived ones; however, in at least one case, the parameter studied varied with lifespan only when related to metabolic rate.

6. The cross-linking of collagen steadily increases with age and it has been known for many years that such cross-linking is very much faster in short-lived rodents than in humans. Bovine skin collagen becomes cross-linked at an intermediate rate.

7. It has been evident for many years that neoplastic transformation occurs much more rapidly in mouse or rat cells than in human cells. This must mean that human cells are better able to maintain their normal phenotype and that rodent cells, in contrast, are relatively unstable in this respect [9].

8. A DNA maintenance methylase is responsible for the inheritance of the pattern of cytosine methylation in DNA. Primary human cells maintain methylation effectively (although it does gradually decline during the *in vitro* lifespan of human fibroblasts), whereas primary mouse cells rapidly lose methylation, and Syrian hamster cells are intermediate. Studies on tissue methylation also demonstrate differences (mouse and humans) during ageing. Also, there is evidence that the epigenetic reactivation of the inactive X chromosome occurs with much greater frequency in mouse somatic cells than human ones. Both this and the preceding point indicate that epigenetic controls need to be much tighter in long-lived mammalian species.

Taken together, these studies strongly support the view that maintenance mechanisms are more effective in longer-lived mammalian species than in short-lived ones; however, with modern techniques many more comparative studies could be carried out. This may be the best way to gain insight into the relation between maintenance, failure of maintenance and the aetiology of age-associated disease.

THE EVOLUTION AND MODULATION OF LONGEVITY

In mammals we see a 30–50-fold range in maximum longevities. What determines these very different lifespans? We can be fairly sure that in mammalian evolution there were trends to increase longevity and also trends to reduce it. The increase is exemplified by the primates, where small lemurs, lorises and small monkeys have a lifespan of 12–15 years, whereas larger species live 30–40 years, the great apes 50–60 years and humans significantly longer. This evolutionary increase in longevity is also associated with slower development times. Carnivores are an example of an evolutionary reduction in longevity. The larger species have a lifespan of about 30 years, whereas the specialised smaller species, such as stoats and weasels, have much shorter lifespans.

Many evolutionary biologists have written extensively on the evolution of ageing, although in most cases the discussion is actually about the evolution of longevities. In a situation where mortality in a natural environment is high, survival depends on rapid growth and reproduction. In contrast, species with a low mortality usually develop and reproduce much more slowly. Imagine a population which is roughly constant with time, with a constant annual mortality in adults. If the mortality increases (for whatever environmental reason), the population is in danger of becoming extinct unless more offspring are produced. Under these circumstances, there will be selection for more rapid growth and reproduction and one would expect the maximum lifespan to decrease. This is what happened in the weasels and stoats, which depend on a constant supply of food, mature very quickly and reproduce rapidly, in comparison to larger carnivores. When annual mortality decreases, the reverse trend is seen. Those females which survive longest will produce, on average, the most offspring and will be fittest in Darwinian terms. Under these circumstances, there can be selection for slower development, later reproduction and longer lifespan, which happened during the evolution of *Homo sapiens* [10]. It has been shown experimentally in *Drosophila* that continual selection of late-breeding females leads to a highly significant increase in lifespan [11].

Evolutionary changes in lifespan are, of course, extremely slow and no doubt involve mutations in multiple genes. These can effect not only obvious phenotypic changes – the province of taxonomists – but also more subtle changes in the efficiency of maintenance, and the relative proportions of total resources invested in reproduction and in preservation of the soma. The expectation is that there is an inverse relation between maximum lifespan and reproductive potential, that is, the maximum number of offspring which could be produced under ideal conditions during an adult female's period of fertility. Good data on longevities and reproduction are harder to obtain from the literature than might be expected. Information on 47 mammalian genera shows that there is indeed a very strong inverse relation between maximum longevity and reproductive potential [1, 12].

Many attempts have been made to relate metabolic rate, animal size or brain size, or combinations of these, with longevities [4, 5]. Although broad relations may exist, there are usually striking exceptions. For example, many bats have a high metabolic rate and an unexceptional brain size, but very long lifespans. They fit well into the reproduction versus longevity relation because they breed very slowly, producing only one or two offspring per year. It is not a surprise that their specialised lifestyle (flight and hanging from the roof of a cave) is associated with a mortality rate which is very much lower than ground-living mammals of comparable size.

Within one species it is important to know how much longevity can be modulated by environmental conditions. The best known example, which has been confirmed many times in rats and mice, is the effect of calorie restriction on longevity. This can be increased by up to 50% if the calorie intake is reduced to 50–60% of the *ad libitum* diet. Moreover, major age-related pathologies are also delayed in these animals. There are severe side-effects of calorie restriction and in particular, the animals become very infertile or sterile. It seems likely that the effect of reduced diet is a natural adaptation to real environments (as opposed to the uniform environment of an animal house). Thus, during a period when there is little available food, reproduction is shut down, resources being diverted instead to preservation of the body until an increased food supply again allows reproduction. It has been shown experimentally that calorie-deprived rats, when provided with a full diet, can reproduce at a much later age than animals fed *ad libitum* throughout life. As well as changes in diet, removal of the anterior pituitary (hypophysectomy) of rats can significantly delay age-related changes and increase longevity [13]. It is not known whether reduced calorie intake significantly increases human lifespan. This information should eventually come from longitudinal studies in which lifestyle parameters are monitored over a considerable proportion of the total lifespan. There is at present a large literature on the environmental effects on human longevity, unsubstantiated by any serious investigations.

In general, we might expect that changes in lifestyle, diet or hormone levels modulate lifespan within a fairly narrow range. As well as molecular or cellular changes, which alter physiological homeostasis, there appears to be a reverse effect in which physiological changes can influence cells and tissues, probably via regulatory pathways. This is far removed from the speculative concept of a neuroendocrine 'pacemaker', which in some way controls overall lifespan.

AGE-ASSOCIATED DISEASE AND THE URGENCY OF RESEARCH ON AGEING

Improvements in health care in this century have resulted in a dramatic increase in the expectation of life, especially in developed countries. This has been achieved at considerable cost, because so many elderly people depend on expensive medical treatment. The expense of health care as a percentage of gross national product doubled between 1960 and 1986 [14] and is set to double again in the first and second decade of the next century. This rate of increase obviously cannot be sustained indefinitely. Instead of spending more and more on age-associated disease, ways and means must be found of curtailing or preventing such disease.

It is often supposed by clinicians that natural ageing is distinct from age-associated disease. One reason for this is that everyone ages and dies, but not all old people develop any particular age-associated disease. Thus, dementia in 50 and 60-year-olds is primarily due to Alzheimer's disease, but many older people have quite normal brain function. The case is similar with cardiovascular disease, type II diabetes, carcinomas and so on. Ageing itself is a normal human occurrence and cannot be regarded as a disease. A more relevant question is the extent to which ageing can be regarded as a 'cluster of pathologies' of varying severity. What we see in populations is a rising incidence of many age-associated diseases, so that any one aged individual may have one or more than one disease, or none.

A reasonable way of thinking about this is shown in the idealised distribution curves of Fig. 1.1. Curve A is the distribution of lifespans about

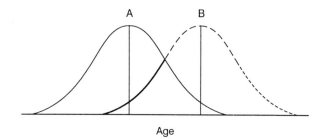

Age

Fig. 1.1 Generalised distribution curves. (A) Longevities of individuals in a country with good health care. (B) The age of diagnosis of a particular age-associated disease. The curves show that only a proportion of individuals develop the disease. The incidence of the disease in the population as a whole increases more than linearly with age (heavy line), and may approximate an exponential increase. The dotted portion of curve B cannot be measured because individuals do not survive long enough (and see text). Reproduced with permission from Robin Holliday in *Understanding Ageing*; published by Cambridge University Press, 1995.

some mean value, which approximates to the expectation of life. Curve B is the distribution at age of diagnosis of a particular age-associated disease. It is always to the right of A. The result is a more than linear increase in this disease in the overall population, but the disease may not develop in very old individuals. In Third World countries where curve A is shifted to the left, fewer people develop the disease. Consider the case of a non-lethal disease, such as loss of sight or hearing, and the hypothetical case of a greatly increased average lifespan. Then curve A becomes similar to curve B or even to the right of it. In this case, everyone in the population would develop the disease.

This situation is to be expected if ageing is multifactorial or multicausal. In one individual, deleterious changes may first affect the cardiovascular system, in another the brain and in a third the lens of the eye, whereas a fourth develops cancer. As was indicated earlier, there is a degree of synchrony in the changes that affect different tissue or organ systems, but this synchrony is only approximate, so the time of onset varies between individuals. It is certainly unrealistic to believe that the various pathologies we are prone to suffer in old age have nothing to do with 'natural ageing', and far more realistic to conclude that these diseases are all components of an overall ageing process.

Vast resources are being devoted worldwide to research into age-associated disease. This research aims to:

- obtain a better understanding of the aetiology or cause of the disease in question;
- develop procedures to prevent or delay the onset of the disease;
- devise better treatments.

The first two are certainly within the province of gerontology. Unfortunately, almost all research is carried out by biomedical scientists who do not believe they are studying any aspect of ageing, nor do specialists in one disease think it is important to be fully aware of research into other age-associated diseases or research into ageing itself. This situation must change because if we are to fully understand the aetiology of each age-associated disease, we need to understand the overall changes that occur during ageing. Gerontology should occupy a central position in biomedical research and not be considered a topic of peripheral interest, as is all too often the case.

This chapter has claimed that we understand the causes of ageing, but this is true only in a broad biological context. In the future, it will be necessary to understand the molecular and cellular details of the many degenerative changes which occur. Table 1.1 lists some of the major failures of maintenance and their consequence in terms of disease. This broad view may be fairly accurate, but of course we need to know in detail all the cellular and molecular changes which occur and why they

Table 1.1 General relations between cell or tissue maintenance and some major human age-associated diseases

Failure of maintenance	Major pathologies
Neurons	Dementias
Retina, lens	Blindness
Insulin metabolism	Type II diabetes
Blood vessels and heart	Cardiovascular and cerebrovascular disease
Bone structure	Osteoporosis
Immune system	Autoimmune disorders
Epigenetic controls	Cancer
Joints	Osteoarthritis
Glomeruli	Renal failure

occur. Only then can effective preventative measures be developed. The first major consequence would be a significant reduction in the costs of health care for the elderly, and therefore a means of curbing the ever-increasing health budget in developed countries. The second consequence would be a significant improvement in the quality of life of the elderly. This would have a third consequence, namely, a reduction in the large number of individuals who at present spend their working lives caring for the infirm elderly, as well as a lessening of the burden too often imposed on younger relatives. The benefits to society as a whole would be immeasurable.

REFERENCES

1. Holliday, R. (1995) *Understanding Ageing*. Cambridge University Press, Cambridge.
2. Medawar, P.B. (1952) *An Unsolved Problem in Biology*. Lewis, London. Reprinted in Medawar P.B. (1981) *The Uniqueness of the Individual*, Dover, New York.
3. Comfort, A. (1964) *Ageing: The Biology of Senescence*, 2nd Ed. Routledge & Kegan Paul, London.
4. Comfort, A. (1979) *The Biology of Senescence*, 3rd Ed. Churchill Livingstone, London.
5. Finch, C.E. (1990) *Longevity, Senescence and the Genome*. University Press, Chicago.
6. Holliday, R. (1996) The urgency of research on ageing. *BioEssays* **18**, 89–90.
7. Lindahl, T. (1993) Instability and decay of the primary structure of DNA. *Nature* **362**, 709–715.
8. Tice, R.R. & Setlow, R.B. (1985) DNA repair and replication in aging organisms and cells. In *Handbook of the Biology of Aging*, 2nd Ed. Eds C.E. Finch & E.L. Schneider, pp. 173–224, Van Nostrand Reinhold, New York.
9. Holliday, R. (1996) Neoplastic transformation: the contrasting stability of human and mouse cells. In *Genetic Instability in Cancer*. Ed. T. Lindahl, pp. 103–115, *Cancer Surveys*, **18**, Cold Spring Harbor Laboratory Press, New York.

10. Holliday, R. (1996) The evolution of human longevity. *Perspect. Biol. Med.* **40,** 100–107.
11. Rose, M.R. (1991) *Evolutionary Biology of Aging.* Oxford University Press, Oxford.
12. Holliday, R. (1994) Longevity and fecundity in eutherian mammals. In *Genetics and Evolution of Aging.* Eds M.R. Rose & C.E. Finch, pp. 217–225, Kluwer Academic Publishers, The Netherlands.
13. Everitt, A.V., Seedsman, N.J. & Jones, F. (1980) The effects of hypophysectomy and continuous food restriction on collagen ageing, proteinuria, incidence of pathology and longevity in the male rat. *Mech. Age Devel.* **12,** 161–172.
14. World Health Organization (1991) *World Health Statistics,* p. 10. WHO, Geneva.

2

Pharmacokinetics of psychotropic drugs in the elderly

Robin A. Braithwaite

INTRODUCTION

The proportion of elderly people (over 65 years of age) in the UK population is steadily rising, being currently 15% (8.5 million persons). This trend will continue into the next century and by the year 2025 it is estimated that there will be around 11 million elderly individuals. Moreover, the proportion of those aged 85 years or more is likely to increase by more than 50%. It is well known that the elderly suffer from more medical and psychiatric problems than younger patients. In particular it has been calculated that the prevalence of mental illness in the elderly in the USA is about 12%, which exceeds that of any other age group. As a consequence, the elderly, particularly the elderly mentally ill, commonly receive multiple medications with the consequent risks of adverse drug reactions and toxicity. There is also a general clinical impression that the elderly are both more 'sensitive' to drugs and suffer from an increased incidence of adverse reactions compared with younger patients. In an extensive early study reported by Hurwitz [1] in Belfast on more than 1000 in-patients, the overall rate of adverse drug reactions was 10% compared with a rate of 15% in patients aged over 60 and 20% in patients over 70 years. Studies on out-patients have also shown a similar picture. Learoyd [2] reported that of 236 consecutive admissions to a psychogeriatric unit, 16% were due to adverse reactions to psychotropic drugs.

Psychopharmacology of Cognitive and Psychiatric Disorders in the Elderly. Edited by David Wheatley and David Smith. Published in 1998 by Chapman and Hall, London. ISBN 0 412 82470 1

More recent studies have confirmed these early observations concerning adverse reactions to psychotropic drugs in the elderly. Ray and co-workers in the USA [3] have shown an increase in the risk of hip fractures following psychotropic drug use in elderly persons and that the risk increased in relation to the dose prescribed. In a subsequent report [4], the risk of motor vehicle crashes was investigated in elderly drivers in relation to psychotropic drug usage. The increased risk of injurious crash involvement was particularly associated with benzodiazepines and cyclic antidepressants. Moreover, the risk increased with dose, being substantial for high doses, and alcohol use was not a confounding factor.

ROLE OF PHARMACOKINETICS

The apparent increase in drug response may be due to an impairment in drug handling, so-called **pharmacokinetic** changes, and/or changes in the number or sensitivity of drug-receptor sites, so-called **pharmacodynamic** changes. A schematic representation of the major pharmacokinetic events following drug administration and the relation with pharmacodynamics is shown in Fig. 2.1. Put more simply, pharmacokinetics is concerned with what the body does to a drug, whereas pharmacodynamics is concerned with what the drug does to the body. There is good evidence that both types of modification take place as part of the ageing process and it may often be difficult to decide the relative importance of

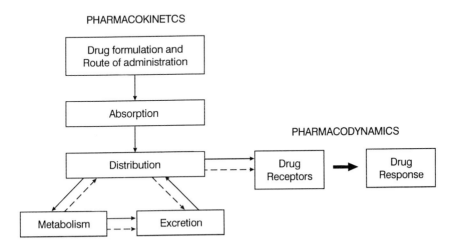

Fig. 2.1 Simplified scheme of pharmacokinetics and pharmacodynamics. (---) Metabolites.

each type of modification. Unfortunately, pharmacodynamic changes have received much less attention than those involving pharmacokinetics. When designing study protocols it would be better to combine the investigation of both pharmacokinetic and pharmacodynamic parameters, following both single and chronic dosing studies.

The main role of pharmacokinetics is to provide a mathematical basis for the description and prediction of the time course of drugs and their metabolites in the body. It is the interindividual variation in pharmacokinetic parameters which determines the concentration of drug (and metabolites) at the receptor site(s) that, in turn, influences the duration of drug action. Pharmacokinetic investigations play an important part in new drug development in phase I and II studies. They are also of value in understanding drug disposition in patients and the influence of age, sex, disease states and environmental factors.

Pharmacokinetic parameters

A number of important pharmacokinetic parameters may be calculated from dosing studies. These commonly include distribution volume (Vd), elimination half-life (t½), area under curve (AUC), clearance (CL) and bioavailability (F).

Distribution volume (Vd)

The distribution volume relates the amount of drug in the body to the concentration of drug in plasma or blood. There are several ways in which Vd may be calculated and has units of L or L kg^{-1} body weight from the ratio of the amount of drug in the body to the plasma concentration.

Half-life (t½)

The half-life is the time taken for the amount of drug in the body, or plasma drug concentration, to reduce its concentration by one-half and can be described by the equation:

$$t\frac{1}{2} = \frac{0.693 \, Vd}{CL} \quad (h)$$

Half-life is directly proportional to distribution volume (Vd), but inversely proportional to drug clearance (CL). The half-life of a drug will be increased as a consequence of an **increase** in distribution volume (Vd) or a **decrease** in clearance (CL). Also, the time taken to reach steady-state plasma concentrations is proportional to the drug elimination half-life; 94% of the steady-state concentration will be reached in four half-lives, following continuous dosing.

Clearance (CL)

Clearance of a drug from the body is additive:

CL systemic = CL renal + CL hepatic + CL other

At steady state, the rate of drug clearance will be equal to the rate of drug administration (assuming that the drug is completely bioavailable) and can be described by the equation:

$$CL = \frac{Dose}{AUC} \; (L \; h^{-1})$$

where AUC is the total area under the plasma drug concentration time curve. Clearance is a much more important parameter than half-life and its significance is often undervalued.

Steady-state concentration (C_{ss})

The average steady-state plasma drug concentration will be reached following multiple dosing and can be described by the equation:

$$C_{ss} = \frac{F.dose}{CL.\tau} \; (\mu g \; L^{-1})$$

where F is the fraction of each dose that is bioavailable (i.e. reaches the systemic circulation), CL the clearance and τ the dosage interval. Thus, if drug clearance is reduced, steady-state drug concentrations will be increased.

There are a number of well-known physiological changes that take place with ageing, which are capable of modifying certain pharmacokinetic parameters in a particular way [5]. The most important of these changes, along with their pharmacokinetic consequences that apply to psychotropic drugs, are summarised in Table 2.1.

DRUG ABSORPTION

There are a number of physiological changes which might at first sight be expected to influence drug absorption. These are a decrease in gastric acid with a subsequent increase in gastric pH, reductions in splanchnic blood flow, gut motility and the rate of gastric emptying. Reduced gastric acid production in the elderly has been shown to reduce the rate of hydrolysis of prodrugs such as the benzodiazepine clorazepate, which is converted to nordiazepam in the stomach. The absorption of a number of dietary constituents such as galactose, calcium, iron and thiamine is known to be reduced in the elderly, but these are all absorbed by active transport mechanisms. The majority of drugs are, however, absorbed by a process of passive diffusion and would therefore not be influenced in the

Table 2.1 Age-related physiological changes affecting drug pharmacokinetics

Process	Altered physiological function	Consequence
Absorption	Reduced gastric acid production Reduced gastric emptying Reduced gastrointestinal motility Reduced splanchnic blood flow Reduced absorptive surface of gut	No consistent changes reported, but may reduce the rate of absorption of some drugs
Distribution	Reduced total body mass (particularly very old)	Increase in dose per unit body weight
	Reduced lean body mass Increase in proportion of fat Reduced body water	*Water-soluble drugs:* Increase in blood levels Reduction in distribution volume
		Lipid-soluble drugs: Reduction in blood levels Increase in distribution volume
	Reduced plasma albumin	Reduced plasma binding and increase in 'free' fraction
	Increased disease-induced acute phase Proteins (e.g α_1-acid glycoprotein)	Increased plasma binding and reduced free fraction
Elimination Renal	Reduced renal blood flow Reduced GFR Reduced tubular secretion	Reduced excretion of water-soluble drugs and polar metabolites
Hepatic	Reduced liver mass Reduced liver blood flow Reduced enzymatic capacity?	Reduced hepatic clearance Increased first-pass bioavailability of some drugs

GFR: glomerular filtration rate

same way [5]. Although only a relatively small number of drugs has been studied so far, the results indicate that drug absorption in the elderly appears to be relatively unimpaired [6]. Although high plasma drug concentrations have sometimes been observed in elderly patients following the oral administration of some drugs, this is probably due to differences in drug distribution or first-pass elimination rather than absorption. Those drugs, however, which might be slowly absorbed along the length of the gut could be influenced by changes in gut transit times caused by constipation or the use of laxatives, in the elderly.

DRUG DISTRIBUTION

Body composition undergoes a number of important changes with the ageing process which can have a marked influence on drug distribution. The elderly, particularly the very old, tend to weigh less than younger patients and the use of standard dosage regimens will, as a consequence, result in generally higher blood and tissue concentrations of drugs. As patients get older, total body water tends to decline. There is also an increase in adipose tissue and a reduction in lean body mass [5]. Thus, the result of such changes in body composition may vary according to the type of drug used. With lipid-soluble drugs, which include many of the psychotropic drugs in common use, such as tricyclic antidepressants, selective serotonin reuptake inhibitors (SSRIs) and benzodiazepines, there will be a relative distribution of drug into fatty tissues so that blood and plasma concentrations will tend to be lower and distribution volumes larger [6–9]. As a direct result of any increase in distribution volume, there will be an increase in the elimination half-life. In the case of water-soluble polar compounds, such as alcohol and lithium, the opposite situation will arise and there will be a trend towards higher blood and plasma concentrations, smaller distribution volumes and shorter half-lives.

A reduction in cardiac output in the elderly may also lead to changes in tissue perfusion and so alter the rate of drug distribution. The main consequence of this may be in intravenous drug administration, such as in the induction of anaesthesia [6].

PLASMA PROTEIN BINDING

Another important factor influencing the distribution of drugs is plasma protein binding. It is the free unbound fraction of the drug in plasma that is 'pharmacologically active' and in direct equilibrium with drug receptor sites. Any alteration in the proportion of drug bound to plasma proteins may, therefore, have important pharmacological consequences. Although plasma albumin declines with age, and may be reduced in disease states common in the elderly or with malnutrition, the concentration of other plasma proteins, particularly 'acute-phase' proteins, may actually increase [6]. Many psychotropic drugs are highly bound to plasma proteins but the binding affinity to albumin may be weak. It has been shown that a number of 'basic' drugs (including several psychotropic drugs) are strongly bound to acute-phase reactant proteins, such as α_1-acid glycoprotein, and studies have shown that the plasma concentration of this protein increases as a consequence of various disease states, such as trauma, infection, cancer and inflammatory disease, which are all common in the elderly [6]. This can lead to an increase in the plasma protein binding of those drugs which have a high affinity for this protein. The presence of multiple disease states is very common in the elderly and likely to be associated with increased plasma concentrations of α_1-acid glycoprotein. The influence of age and the presence of multiple disease states is, therefore, going to lead to a complicated situation with regard to overall changes in plasma protein binding and one where simple predictions cannot be made.

Moreover, any change in free drug concentration may be offest by a change in free drug clearance.

DRUG ELIMINATION

Renal excretion

Glomerular filtration rate (GFR) is reduced in the elderly, there being an average decline in function of some 35% between the ages of 20 and 90 years [5]. Also, renal blood flow, tubular secretion and urine concentrating ability during water deprivation all decline with age. It is therefore possible to show that there is some impairment in the clearance of water-soluble drugs or polar metabolites, whose chief route of elimination is via the kidney [6]. Lithium is the best known psychotropic drug to be eliminated through the kidney, and intoxication may be complicated by renal insufficiency or fluid and electrolyte imbalance.

Hepatic elimination

The majority of psychotropic drugs are eliminated from the body by oxidative metabolism in the hepatic microsomal enzyme system (cytochrome p450 isoenzymes). In the elderly there are reductions in hepatic mass, liver blood flow and possibly enzyme activity, which are all likely to lead to some impairment in the body's ability to metabolise drugs [5,6].

The hepatic clearance of a drug (CLH) is related to organ extraction (E) and liver blood flow (Q) by the equation:

$$CLH = Q.E$$

For high extraction drugs (E > 0.7), such as tricyclic antidepressants, CLH will be strongly influenced by liver blood flow and any reduction in flow will lead to reduced extraction and a large reduction in first-pass elimination, producing much higher drug concentrations. In contrast, if E is small (< 0.3) CLH will be largely influenced by hepatic extraction and relatively independent of liver blood flow.

In a number of early studies plasma elimination half-life was used as an index of drug metabolism, but this is misleading as half-life may just as easily be influenced by changes in distribution volume as by changes in clearance. A clear indication that the elderly have some impairment in the ability to metabolise drugs came from early studies by O'Malley and co-workers [10] on antipyrene. It was shown that antipyrene plasma half-life was 50% longer and its clearance 40% reduced in elderly subjects compared with younger controls. There are now data on a number of other drugs where similar findings have been observed, but the overall picture is far from clear and conflicting findings have been reported for some drugs. Study design and patient selection are important factors that have led to much of the conflict in findings, particularly concerning drug elimination in the elderly [6,8,9].

BENZODIAZEPINES

The elderly are generally considered to be more 'sensitive' to benzodiazepines than younger patients. This is thought to be due to either pharmacokinetic or pharmacodynamic age-related changes or a combination of both factors [7,8]. The majority of benzodiazepines, particularly those with long elimination half-lives (e.g. diazepam), are metabolised by hepatic microsomal oxidative enzymes whereas others may be eliminated by glucuronide conjugation (e.g. oxazepam, temazepam) and others less commonly by nitroreduction (e.g. nitrazepam) [8].

The effect of age on the pharmacokinetics of the benzodiazepine group of drugs, particularly diazepam, has been investigated in more detail than perhaps any other group of psychotropic drugs [7,8]. Early studies reported by Klotz and co-workers [11] on diazepam showed that its plasma half-life was prolonged in the elderly and that its distribution volume was also increased, but there was no significant reduction in drug clearance. In more detailed studies carried out by Greenblatt and co-workers [8] the influence of other factors, such as sex, protein binding and cigarette smoking, was also assessed. These studies showed that diazepam half-life was prolonged in both elderly males and females; however, distribution volume was larger in females than in males regardless of age, and larger in the elderly regardless of sex [8]. Diazepam plasma protein binding was also reduced in the elderly, mainly as a consequence of reduced albumin concentrations [8]. The clearance of unbound 'free' diazepam tended to be higher in females than in males of both young and old subjects, and was higher in the young than in the elderly of both sexes. Smoking was also associated with higher clearance values. More recently, the pharmacokinetics of diazepam have been studied by Herman and Wilkinson [12] in small groups of young and elderly subjects, following both single and repeated oral dosing. No age-related reduction in clearance or increase in steady-state concentration was observed, although half-lives were increased twofold in elderly subjects due to an increase in distribution volume. The consequence of an increased elimination half-life is that steady-state plasma concentrations will be attained more slowly and decay more slowly following cessation of dosage compared with younger patients. An interesting recent study of the sensitivity to triazolam in the elderly investigated both pharmacokinetic and pharmacodynamic changes [13]. Triazolam caused a significantly greater impairment of psychomotor performance in healthy elderly subjects compared with younger subjects. The reported effects were caused by reduced drug clearance, leading to higher plasma concentrations of triazolam, rather than any increased sensitivity to the drug. Therefore, a 50% reduction dosage in elderly subjects has been recommended for this drug [13].

With such a complex situation it is perhaps difficult to generalise to the situation with other benzodiazepines. It would seem that for those benzodiazepines which undergo oxidative metabolic transformations (e.g. diazepam, chlordiazepoxide, flurazepam), clearances may not necessarily be reduced, but drug half-lives are increased because distribution volumes are increased. For those benzodiazepines which undergo simple glucuronide conjugation (e.g. oxazepam, temazepam and lorazepam), the ageing process appears to exert only a minimal influence on drug clearance.

NON-BENZODIAZEPINE HYPNOTICS AND ANXIOLYTICS

Buspirone

Buspirone is a relatively new non-benzodiazepine anxiolytic. Preliminary studies following single and repeated dose studies in young and elderly volunteer subjects have found no difference in pharmacokinetic parameters [6].

Zopiclone

Zopiclone is a non-benzodiazepine hypnotic agent that is now widely prescribed. It is marketed as a racemic mixture of R- and S- isomers which undergo stereoselective metabolism. Plasma concentrations of the S- isomer are much higher than the R- isomer. The S- isomer has a lower distribution volume and lower clearance compared with its R- isomer [14]. Preliminary studies indicate that elderly individuals show much higher (total) plasma zopiclone and metabolite concentrations than young healthy volunteers [14]. These changes are probably due to reductions in both renal and hepatic clearance in elderly subjects, but further studies are needed to explore the clinical consequences of the pharmacokinetic changes in more detail.

ANTIDEPRESSANTS

Tricyclic antidepressants

The pharmacokinetics of tricyclic antidepressants in relation to age has been investigated over many years and a large number of studies has been reported and extensively reviewed [6,9]. Most studies have concerned amitriptyline, nortriptyline, imipramine and desipramine and relatively few concern other tricyclics such as dothiepin and clomipramine. The available evidence suggests that the clearance of some tricyclic antidepressants is reduced in the elderly and that half-lives may also be increased [6,9]. Many studies, however, have suffered from problems of study design, particularly the lack of inclusion of younger control groups and the influence of concurrent disease states [6,9]. Most studies have shown that there is a large interindividual variation in steady-state plasma drug concentrations in all patients receiving similar doses of tricyclic antidepressant, which is apparent even in younger healthy patients. This 'variability' appears to increase in the elderly, although some of the reported changes may well be due to concurrent physical illness rather than age itself [15]. There is clear evidence that some elderly patients, particularly those with concurrent illness, have a significantly reduced drug clearance and increased elimination half-life. There is also evidence that the renal clearance of hydroxylated metabolites of antidepressants, some of which are pharmacologically active, may be reduced in the elderly [6].

An interesting investigation of the influence of age and concurrent disease states on the pharmacokinetics of tricyclic antidepressants was carried out by Dawling and co-workers [6] in a series of studies in patients aged between 68 and 100 years. Patients were suffering from a variety of physical disorders, but were also sufficiently depressed to warrant treatment with a tricyclic antidepressant drug, and were given single and repeated doses of nortriptyline. The plasma elimination half-life and total oral clearance of nortriptyline in these patients was significantly different from that observed in young healthy volunteers in previous studies. The patient group differed from the young control group not only in age and sex distribution, but also because the subjects were hospitalised, suffering from various physical disorders and receiving treatment with a wide variety of drugs. For these reasons, the difference in nortriptyline pharmacokinetics between the two groups was probably only partly due to age differences, and the presence of physical illness and medication may have been equally important [6]. These studies were also able to demonstrate that 'high' plasma drug concentrations could be predicted from single point drug concentrations observed following the administration of a standardised single oral dose of drug. Monitoring of steady-state antidepressant concentrations or simple pharmacokinetic dosage prediction tests may be a useful way of avoiding toxicity in elderly patients, particularly those who are frail or have concurrent physical illness.

Trazodone

This novel antidepressant has been in clinical use for many years. It has fewer cholinergic side-effects compared with tricyclic antidepressants and is commonly prescribed to elderly patients. Studies suggest that its clearance is reduced in the elderly, particularly in the case of elderly men; also elderly men and women appear to have larger distribution volumes and as a consequence longer half-lives [9].

Selective serotonin reuptake inhibitors (SSRIs)

Age-related changes in the pharmacokinetics of several SSRI drugs have now been reported, but the situation is complex, there being important differences in the pharmacokinetics between members of this relatively new class of antidepressant drug [16,17]. These changes have important implications concerning the incidence of adverse effects and interaction between SSRIs and some concomitantly prescribed medications.

An age-related increase in plasma drug concentrations has been reported for citalopram, paroxetine, fluoxetine and sertraline; no change has been reported for fluvoxamine [16]. The situation is more complex in the case of citalopram and fluoxetine, which are marketed as racemic mixtures which will undergo stereospecific metabolism. Thus, fluoxetine (R- and S- isomers) will produce R- and S-norfluoxetine. It is important to note that R- and S-fluoxetine and S-norfluoxetine are of similar potency regarding inhibition of serotonin uptake, whereas R-norfluoxetine is much less potent [16].

The SSRIs have all been shown to be inhibitors of hepatic microsomal cytochrome (CYP) enzymes concerned with drug metabolism [16]. There are several isoforms of these enzymes and SSRIs vary in their inhibition of particular CYP isoenzymes. Citalopram and sertraline appear to be weak inhibitors of CYP 2D6 isoenzyme, whereas fluvoxamine, fluoxetine and paroxetine are potent inhibitors of several different CYP isoenzymes, including CYP 2D6. There is therefore a strong potential for drug–drug pharmacokinetic interactions, particularly in elderly patients, where the clearance of concomitantly prescribed drugs such as theophylline, tricyclic antidepressants and warfarin may be significantly impaired [16].

Lithium

The prophylactic use of lithium in the elderly appears to be associated with a high incidence of side-effects, particularly neurotoxicity [18]. The clearance of lithium is reduced in the elderly and there is also a correlation between the renal clearance of lithium and creatinine clearance. The elderly also appear to require smaller doses of lithium to achieve the same therapeutic control as younger patients, but it is unclear if this is due to pharmacokinetic or pharmacodynamic changes [18]. A reduction in lithium maintenance dose is clearly indicated in the elderly, particularly for those patients with renal impairment or receiving concurrent medication that may influence fluid and electrolyte balance. Single dose pharmacokinetic tests, using a single drug measurement, can be used to predict lithium dosage requirements in such patients.

ALCOHOL

Although studies suggest that the elderly consume less alcohol than younger members of the population, the influence of age on the pharmacokinetics of alcohol has been poorly investigated. In a study of healthy males (aged 21–81 years) the elimination rate of alcohol was not influenced by age [19]. However, higher peak blood alcohol concentrations were seen in the elderly, probably due to a decrease in distribution volume (Vd) caused by a reduction in lean body mass [19]. A reduction in first-pass metabolism of alcohol with ageing in males but not females has also been reported, but further work is required to confirm the clinical significance of this observation.

NEUROLEPTIC DRUGS

There is a surprising lack of information regarding the influence of age on the pharmacokinetics of this large disparate group of drugs. It is likely that the situation for some drugs will be similar to that of tricyclic antidepressants.

CONCLUSION

It is clear that there is no consistent pattern of change with regard to pharmacokinetics and ageing. There are surprisingly large gaps in our knowledge concerning the pharmacokinetics of many common psychotopic drugs used in elderly patients. The disposition of some drugs may be impaired (reduced clearance) in some elderly patients, which may be the cause of increased drug sensitivity. It can be very difficult to separate the relative influence of ageing (chronological or biological) from the presence of multiple disease states, environmental factors such as medication, diet and the use of tobacco and alcohol. Thus, in the absence of any simple guide, each drug should be individually investigated using appropriate pharmacokinetic studies. At the same time, it is important not to lose sight of the possible importance of pharmacodynamic changes in the elderly [20,21]. Homeostasis in general becomes less responsive with age, so the elderly may be more susceptible to drug toxicity than younger patients [22]. Our understanding of pharmacodynamic changes in the elderly is extremely limited as is the relation between drug concentration and clinical response. Single dose pharmacokinetic studies are not always helpful in elucidating the effect of ageing on drug handling. Chronic dosing studies on larger populations of both young and old patients are much more meaningful. It may not always be possible to carry out traditional pharmacokinetic measurements that require invasive dosing studies or the collection of large numbers of specimens. A small number of blood specimens collected from a large population of patients over time during chronic dosing may give invaluable information and foresight of pharmacokinetic changes. Such studies should include the measurement of parent drug and active metabolite concentrations, also individual isomers where the drug is given as a racemic mixture. Combined pharmacokinetic and pharmacodynamic studies are also likely to be of greater value in deciding the clinical consequences of any change in drug handling, particularly when dealing with complex issues such as psychotropic drug abuse and dependency [23]. It would also be valuable to include more elderly patients in clinical trials in the early development of new psychotropic drugs [24].

It follows that extra care should be taken with the elderly in the choice of an appropriate drug, its formulation and dosage regimen. As a general rule the elderly may sometimes require smaller doses than are customarily given to younger patients, reflecting the slow decline in body function with age. No simple generalisations can be made regarding the influence of age alone on pharmacokinetics but special caution is required in the treatment of very frail or infirm elderly patients who may require greatly reduced drug dosages and who otherwise may be at risk of accumulating excessive drug concentrations, leading to overdosage and toxicity. The best recommendation is to start with a low dose and titrate up to the lowest effective dose, or the appearance of side-effects.

ACKNOWLEDGEMENTS

I thank Mrs D. Woolley for secretarial assistance in the preparation of this manuscript. Also Dr Robin Ferner for helpful comments and criticism.

REFERENCES

1. Hurwitz, N. (1969) Predisposing factors in adverse reactions to drugs. *Br. Med. J.* **1**, 536–540.
2. Learoyd, B.M. (1972) Psychotropic drugs and the elderly patient. *Med. J. Aust.* **1**, 1131–1133.
3. Ray, W.A., Griffin, M.R., Schaffner, W. *et al.* (1987) Psychotropic drug abuse and the risk of hip fracture. *N. Engl. J. Med.* **316**, 363–369.
4. Ray, W.A., Fought, R.L. and Decker, M.D. (1992) Psychoactive drugs and risk of injurious motor vehicle crashes in elderly drivers. *Am. J. Epidemiol.* **136**, 873–883.
5. Ritschel, W.A. (1988) *Gerontokinetics – the Pharmacokinetics of Drugs in the Elderly.* Telford Press, Caldwell, N.J.
6. Dawling, S. and Crome, P. (1989) Clinical pharmacokinetic considerations in the elderly. An update. *Clin. Pharmacokinet.* **17**, 236–263.

7. Greenblatt, D.J., Shader, R.I. and Harmatz, J.S. (1989) Implications of altered drug disposition in the elderly: studies of benzodiazepines. *J. Clin. Pharmacol.* **29**, 866–872.
8. Greenblatt, D.J., Harmatz, J.S. and Shader, R.I. (1991) Clinical pharmacokinetics of anxiolytics and hypnotics in the elderly. Therapeutic considerations (part I). *Clin. Pharmacokinet.* **21**, 165–177.
9. Von Moltke, L.L., Greenblatt, D.J. and Shader, R.I. (1993) Clinical pharmacokinetics of antidepressants in the elderly. Therapeutic implications. *Clin. Pharmacokinet.* **24**, 141–160.
10. O'Malley, K., Crooks, J., Duke, E. and Stephenson, I.H. (1971) Effect of age and sex on human drug metabolism. *Br. Med. J.* III, 607–609.
11. Klotz, U., Avant, G.R., Hoyumpa, A. *et al.* (1975) The effect of age and liver disease on the disposition and elimination of diazepam in adult man. *J. Clin. Invest.* **55**, 347–359.
12. Herman, R.J. and Wilkinson, G.R. (1996) Disposition of diazepam in young and elderly subjects after acute and chronic dosing. *Br. J. Clin. Pharmacol.* **42**, 147–155.
13. Greenblatt, D.J., Harmatz., J.S., Shapiro, L. *et al.* (1991) Sensitivity to triazolam in the elderly. *N. Engl. J. Med.* **324**, 169–168.
14. Galliot, J., Le Roux, Y., Houghton G.W. *et al.* (1987) Clinical factors for pharmacokinetics of zopiclone in the elderly and in patients with liver and renal insufficiency. *Sleep* **10** (Suppl. 1), 7–21.
15. Braithwaite, R.A., Montgomery, S.A. and Dawling, S. (1979) Age, depression and tricyclic aptidepressant levels. In: *Drugs and the Elderly – Perspectives in Geriatric Clinical Pharmacology*, ed. J. Crooks and I.H Stevenson. Macmillan, London, pp. 133–143.
16. Preskorn, S.H. (1997) Clinically relevant pharmacology of selective serotonin reuptake inhibitors – an overview with emphasis on pharmacokinetics and effects on oxidative drug metabolism. *Clin. Pharmacokinet.* **32** (Suppl. 1), 1–21.
17. Ronfield, R.A., Tremaine, L.M. and Wilner, K. (1997) Pharmacokinetics of sertraline and its N-desmethyl metabolite in elderly and young male and female volunteers. *Clin. Pharmacokinet.* **32** (Suppl. 1), 22–30.
18. Hardy, B.G., Shulman, K.I., Mackenzie, S.E. *et al.* (1987) Pharmacokinetics of lithium in the elderly. *J. Clin. Psychopharmacol.* **7**, 153–158.
19. Vestal, R.E., McGuire, E.A., Tobin, J.D. *et al.* (1977) Ageing and ethanol metabolism. *Clin. Pharmacol. Ther.* **21**, 343–354.
20. Greenblatt, D.J., Harmatz, J.S. and Shader, R.I. (1991) Clinical pharmacokinetics of anxiolytics and hypnotics in the elderly. Therapeutic considerations (part II). *Clin. Pharmacokinet.* **21**, 262–273.
21. Jackson, S.H.D. (1994) Pharmacodynamics in the elderly. *J. R. Soc. Med.* **87** (Suppl. 23), 5–7.
22. Swift, C.G. (1990) Pharmacodynamics: changes in homeostatic mechanisms, receptor and target organ sensitivity in the elderly. *Br. Med. Bull.* **46**, 36–52.
23. Özdemir V., Fourie J., Busto U. and Naranjo, C.A. (1996) Pharmacokinetic changes in the elderly – do they contribute to drug abuse and dependence? *Clin. Pharmacokinet.* **31**, 372–385.
24. Crome, P. and Flanagan, R.J. (1994) Pharmacokinetic studies in elderly people, are they necessary? *Clin. Pharmacokinet.* **26**, 243–247.

3

Side-effects of psychotropic drugs

David A. Smith

INTRODUCTION

As mentioned in other chapters of this book, mental illness is quite common in the elderly and, therefore, the prescription of psychotropic drugs is also common. In fact, psychotropic drugs are among the most frequent prescriptions provided to the elderly after cardiovascular medications and analgesics. The prevalence of chronic physical illness and degenerative disorders rises with age, leading to special vulnerabilities among the elderly to the side-effects of psychotropic medications. Table 3.1 lists some age-related conditions that create special risks for the elderly as psychotropic drugs are prescribed [1].

Coupled with these concerns, patient compliance or adherence problems and physician errors such as duplicate therapy and failure to have accurate record of the patient's drug regimen, the vulnerabilities of the elderly lead to frequent adverse drug reactions severe enough to require hospitalization. Most psychiatric care and prescription to elders is provided by primary care physicians; however, the accuracy of diagnosis and the appropriateness of therapeutic choices by these physicians has often been impugned in the literature [2].

These problems became so apparent, even to the lay public, that in the USA patient advocacy groups successfully catalyzed reform legislation which eventually enacted bureaucratic regulations for the use of major and minor tranquilizers in American nursing homes [3,4]. A thorough discussion of these regulations, the science behind them and their effects

Psychopharmacology of Cognitive and Psychiatric Disorders in the Elderly. Edited by David Wheatley and David Smith. Published in 1998 by Chapman and Hall, London. ISBN 0 412 82470 1

Table 3.1 Some age-related
conditions resulting in
increased risks for psy-
chotropic drug side-effects

Arrhythmias
Constipation
Dementia
Diabetes mellitus
Gait disorders
Glaucoma
Hypertension
Hypothermia
Malnutrition
Prostatic hypertrophy
Seizure disorders

---

on American long-term care facilities has been published by Stoudemire and Smith [5]. Problems not easily addressed in regulation remain. Inattendance by the long-term care physician at the bedside and telephone prescription in response to episodic problems, but without later follow-up, are prevalent [6]. Integration of the prescription into the long-term treatment plan, careful diagnosis and objectification of symptoms, followed by an interval review of treatment efficacy seldom occurs. Periodic screening with standardized instruments to assess for side-effects is rare.

Too often, side-effects may go unrecognized altogether or be blamed on other causes. The elderly often hide or fail to volunteer complaints about their physical or mental symptoms. They may believe that these problems are unimportant, not correctable, are due to aging or that no one cares. They may be reluctant to waste the doctor's time or to imply a challenge to his/her authority by insinuating that the treatment is causing a problem. They may not wish to add to others' perceptions of their frailty out of fear that they will be institutionalized, or they may find the complaint itself embarrassing or ego-dystonic, e.g. incontinence, sexual dysfunction, falling, confusion or memory problems.

On the other hand, physicians may subliminally refuse to consider that a treatment they have prescribed with the intent of doing service is having the opposite effect. They may not recognize the slow insidious onset of side-effects from a psychotropic drug with a long elimination half-life, failing to make a temporal connection between these events, especially if the original prescription were made by telephone, as is often the case in long-term care. They may ascribe the symptom to age-related diseases, or to aging itself. Finally, they may simply not know that the psychotropic drug can cause a particular symptom.

NEUROTRANSMITTER EFFECTS AND SIDE-EFFECTS

A listing of each of the psychotropic drug classes followed by a listing of possible side-effects, such as is found in the Physician's Desk Reference or various drug compendiums, would be very redundant and lack pedagogical purpose. Instead, this chapter explains psychotropic drug side-effects by association with neurotransmitter systems and anatomic/physiologic systems. Finally, some additional relevant comments are made about the various drug classes.

The similarities and differences among psychotropic drug classes and the members within each class can largely be explained by neurotransmitter receptor affinities and pharmacodynamics. The astute clinician is wise to choose a few drugs from each class and know the nuances of neurotransmitter action and pharmacodynamics of each. One's personal therapeutic armamentarium may then contain several drugs within each class which are different from each other. The trick of successful prescription of psychotropics is not so much that of choosing the most efficacious drug, as most are very similar in this regard. Rather, it is important to choose a drug for which the side-effect profile best avoids the vulnerabilities of the patient, or in which the side-effects themselves become therapeutic. In the former instance, one would avoid a potent anticholinergic medication in a demented patient presumed to already have a cholinergic deficit, or in a patient prone to urinary retention. In the latter instance, one may choose a tricyclic antidepressant over a selective serotonin uptake inhibitor if the antihistaminic effect of sedation or the blunting of gastric acid secretion is desirable rather than problematic. Table 3.2 lists several (but not all) neurotransmitter systems and associated potential central nervous system (CNS) and systemic side-effects.

PSYCHOTROPIC DRUG SIDE-EFFECTS BY ANATOMIC/PHYSIOLOGIC SYSTEM

Psychotropic drug side-effects may also be considered on the basis of physiologic effect by organ system. The following is such a discussion, with an explanation based on neurotransmitter effects where they are known.

Integumentary

Antipsychotics may cause rash by several mechanisms including cutaneous anaphylaxis (hives) but no known reports of systemic anaphylaxis exist. Other immune-mediated rashes also occur. Dopamine is involved in the synthesis of skin pigmentation and melanosis may occur abnormally in the skin (and also in the retina) of patients treated with antipsychotics, leading to a gray discoloration. This is accentuated by sun exposure.

Table 3.2 Neurotransmitter systems and related central nervous system/systemic side-effects

Anticholinergic	Decreased salivary production
	Decreased sweating
	Decreased gastric acid
	Increased intraocular pressure
	Impaired accommodation and vision
	Urinary retention
	Decreased gastrointestinal motility
	Tachycardia
	Hyperpyrexia
	Impotence
	Retrograde ejaculation
	Psychosis or delirium
Antidopaminergic	Movement disorders
	Tardive
	Extrapyramidal
	Swallowing disorders
	Galactorrhea or amenorrhea
	Gynecomastia
	Pigmentation
Antihistaminic	Sedation
	Hypotension
	Weight gain
	Altered glucagon secretion
Antiserotonergic	Pigmentation
Anti-alpha 1 adrenergic	Arrhythmia and tachycardia
	Angina
	Insomnia
	Tremor
	Impaired glucose metabolism

Other patients will develop photosensitivity and burn easily. Sunscreens and protective clothing are worthwhile. Benzodiazopines cause rash only rarely, while antidepressants of all classes are frequent offenders.

Special senses

Phenothiazines have been implicated in the development of retinopathy and cataract formation. They may induce melanin–phenothiazine complex deposits in the cornea and lens to a degree that will affect vision. A slit-lamp evaluation by an ophthalmologist on an annual basis may be prudent, especially if a phenothiazine is given in high dose over long periods, or if there is hyperpigmentation of the skin.

Any antipsychotic drug with anticholinergic activity may cause blurred vision by interfering with the accommodative reflex. Of course, elderly patients already have an absence of accommodative reflex and are not generally further impaired on this basis. Of greater potential concern, all such drugs may cause pupillary dilatation to the point of narrowing the canal of Schlemm and precipitating an episode of narrow angle glaucoma in susceptible individuals. A history of this type of glaucoma should always be sought before prescribing anticholinergic drugs. Such a history does not absolutely contraindicate use, but necessitates precaution and follow-up. Anticholinergics often cause significant decreased secretions of mucous membranes in the nose and mouth. Epistaxis, tooth decay, halitosis and the discomfort of 'cotton mouth' are possible.

Endocrine

Lithium may induce goiter and hypothyroidism. The elderly appear to be at special risk and may not be as easily recognized when suffering this side-effect. Periodic evaluation of the thyroid with palpation and a thyroid-stimulating hormone (TSH) assay is recommended.

Hyponatremia

Hyponatremia may be caused by a number of psychotropics acting through several different endocrine mechanisms. When developing rapidly or to extremes, especially in susceptible individuals, seizure activity may occur.

The selective serotonin reuptake inhibitors (SSRIs), tricyclics, bupropion and monoamine oxidase inhibitors (MAOIs) have all been implicated in the development of the syndrome of inappropriate antidiuretic hormone release (SIADH). The offending agent causes oversecretion of this pituitary hormone which in turn causes the nephron of the kidney to fail to excrete free water. The serum osmolality is low (diluted) in comparison to the urine osmolality obtained simultaneously. Hypertonic saline infusions are almost never warranted even in patients who suffer seizures. Instead, absolute fluid restriction and discontinuance of the offending drug are the necessary interventions. The development of SIADH may be due to a certain drug, or may recur when the patient is treated with any alternative psychotropic choice.

Hyponatremia may be induced through a sodium-losing nephropathy caused by carbamazepine (Tegretol). If this loss is negligible, it may be ignored. Giving increased dietary salt may be helpful. Hyponatremia may also occur with pathological water drinking in some patients treated with antipsychotics. The mechanism of this disorder is poorly understood. The elderly probably are at less risk than younger patients. Pathological water drinking or polydipsic syndrome is not simply related to dry mouth and the anticholinergic effects of drugs, nor is it under behavioral control. The affected individuals may drink huge quantities of fluids, even neglecting nutrition in favor of water if weight is used as a measure in a behavioral modification intervention. For most patients, homeostatic mechanisms serve to prevent severe hyponatremia and seizure, even if large volumes are consumed. Smokers are at significant risk. Nicotine is a potent stimulator of antidiuretic hormone leading to decreased free-water clearance by the kidney and therefore a much greater potential for dilutional hyponatremia. This author hypothesizes that endorphin receptors are enhanced by hyponatremia and that these individuals may truly be experiencing, as the old terminology expressed, water intoxication.

Conversely, hyp*er*natremia may occasionally be induced by lithium therapy through the mechanism of nephrogenic diabetes insipidus. In certain individuals and at any point in the course of therapy, lithium may render the renal tubule incapable of retaining free water. These individuals require large volumes of fluid to maintain normal serum sodium and osmolality and if denied, will rapidly become profoundly dehydrated. The potential exists to confuse pathological water drinking with lithium-induced nephrogenic diabetes insipidus, with fatal consequences.

Weight and appetite

The antihistaminic activity of many psychotropics, such as phenothiazines and tricyclic antidepressants, increases appetite, decreases glucagon secretion and causes weight gain. To the contrary, two phenothiazines (loxapine and molindone) have been associated with weight loss. Those psychotropics, e.g. tricyclics, that enhance norepinephrine systems increase appetite, particularly for sweets and carbohydrates. Weight gain and loss of control in diabetes may result. Similarly, diabetes may be worsened with beta-blockers as the secretion of insulin from islet cells is under beta-adrenergic control. Dopamine and serotonin are found in pancreatic beta-cells and are probably also involved in insulin release.

Other psychotropics may have the opposite effect on the diabetic patient. Monoamine oxidase inhibitors have been observed to lead to hypoglycemia when combined with oral antidiabetic agents or insulin. Lithium causes an increase in insulin secretion, enhanced peripheral uptake of insulin and improved glucose utilization very similar to the oral antidiabetic agents themselves.

Sexual function

Many psychoactive agents have the potential to cause sexual dysfunction. In elderly patients this may be of less importance due to a pre-existing decline in sexual function or interest, or as the result of loss of a partner; however, for many elders this *is* a significant problem. Erectile and ejaculatory disturbance in males and anorgasmia or libido problems in both sexes may occur with most agents. Trazadone, in particular, may cause increased libido in females and priapism (non-sexually stimulated and unrelenting erections) in males. Highly anticholinergic drugs like thioridazine are especially likely to cause retrograde ejaculation. Mechanisms for sexual dysfunction due to psychotropics include CNS effects, changes in gonadotropins, increased prolactin (particularly with major tranquilizers) and effects on the sympathetic and parasympathetic nervous systems. This constellation of mechanisms leads to a confusing array of possibilities such that a certain drug may have seemingly opposite effects on sexual functions in different patients, and drugs with opposite neurochemical effects may cause the same sexual dysfunction in different patients.

Rather than memorizing a list of possibilities for each drug, the clinician should remain alert to the possibility of sexual dysfunction in elderly patients on psychoactive medication and, when relevant, should actively seek a history of these side-effects on follow-up, as many elders will not volunteer such sensitive information.

Gynecomastia is occasionally seen in men treated with benzodiazepines and antipsychotics. Elevated estradiol and prolactin may explain this phenomenon.

Respiratory system

Any psychotropic drug with potential to sedate could, if taken in overdose, produce hypoventilation or apnea. This is particularly true when sedatives including alcohol are taken in combination. Elders with chronic obstructive pulmonary disease or sleep apnea syndromes are at special risk, and if these conditions are severe, then prescription of sedative drugs is relatively contraindicated. In rare psychiatric emergencies they may be prescribed, but only with adequate monitoring of respiratory status. Hypercarbic patients may appear lethargic, discouraging further sedation, but hypoxic ones often appear agitated, possibly leading to further prescription of sedatives and compounding of the problem. Anticholinergic and antihistaminic drugs can dry secretions. Thickened bronchial secretions could theoretically worsen chronic lung disease and asthma.

Cardiovascular system

Psychotropics may cause hypotension which is either fixed or orthostatic in nature through peripheral alpha-adrenergic blockade, central alpha-adrenergic stimulation or direct vasodilation. The elderly, especially those with hypertension, other cardiovascular diseases, diabetes and those on other vasoactive medications, are prone to orthostasis, defined as a drop of 20 mm Hg or more systolic, or 10 mm Hg in diastolic pressure. Those not meeting these strict criteria, but who complain of lightheadedness on rising, should also be considered as suffering orthostatic hypotension because individual variations in cerebral perfusion relative to blood pressure exist.

Long duration reclining or sitting, dehydration and the post-prandial state increase the risk of symptomatic hypotension. To measure postural changes, the examiner should measure blood pressure on reclining, sitting, immediately on standing and one minute after standing. The latter reading is most likely to demonstrate the abnormality. Hypotension, fixed or postural, may best be treated with a switch to a drug with less alpha-adrenergic affinity, reducing the dose or, when this is not possible, by behavioral interventions. These include sleeping with the head elevated, arising gradually, taking multiple smaller meals, increasing salt and fluids, or by wearing support hose. Occasionally, caffeine, fluorocortisone or sympathomimetics are required. Hypotension induced by psychotropics may be accompanied by reflex tachycardia. Additionally, alpha-adrenergic blockade and increases in circulating catecholamines may cause tachycardia and extra-systoles. Psychotropics with anticholinergic activity may also cause tachycardia by stimulating the sinus node. Monoamine oxidase inhibitors may cause hypertension and hypertensive crises when combined with many other medications or tyramine-containing foods. Sufficient 'washout' periods should always be observed when changing to or from an MAOI drug. The dangers, however, may be overstated in the literature, and many believe that this class of antidepressant drug is underutilized.

Many psychotropic drugs have effects on cardiac conduction. These may be either antiarrhythmic or proarrhythmic. At therapeutic dose, they are, however, almost always negligible even in patients with cardiac disease. The mechanisms involved include negative effects on contractility which could lead to congestive heart failure, increased catecholamines and prolongation of conduction times and refractory periods due to interference with the 'fast' or sodium channel metabolism of cardiac myofibrils. Thus, these drugs, e.g. phenothiazines and tricyclics, are quinidine-like. In overdose, situations where drugs with similar action are used in combination, or in susceptible individuals with a congenital prolongation of the QT interval, an arrhythmia may result. Torsade de pointes ventricular tachycardia may be asymptomatic or progress to ventricular fibrillation and death. A rotating cardiac axis defines this condition. The tracing appears to spiral if one looks at the rhythm strip as if it were three-dimensional. Like quinidine toxicity which presents by the same mechanism, this psychotropic-induced cardiac arrhythmia may, when malignant, require treatment with sodium lactate and a temporary transvenous pacemaker.

Neuroleptics and tricyclic antidepressants may have other less serious effects on cardiac conduction as seen on the electrocardiogram. Increased duration of PR and QRS may occur, whilst T-wave, U-wave and ST segment changes are relatively common. Lithium may also flatten T-waves. While benign, these changes may confuse the clinician, especially when cardiac disease is also present. When in doubt, a repeat ECG in the morning, in the fasting state, may show partial or complete correction of T-wave flattening, confirming that the phenomenon is related to psychotropic drug therapy rather than ischemic heart disease. Ventricular ectopy may be caused or aggravated by chloral hydrate or trazadone, while maprotiline has been implicated in induction of atrial fibrillation.

Care should be exercised in choosing a psychotropic drug for patients with any pre-existing cardiac condition. With the proper choice of agent, monitoring of blood levels and compliance, and examination of the blood pressure, pulse and ECG when the steady state is reached, these risks are slight. No patient should be denied pharmacotherapy for mental illness out of fear of exacerbation of cardiac disease. Certainly, untreated mental illness poses a greater danger for deterioration of cardiovascular status than appropriate psychotropic prescription.

Gastrointestinal and hepatic systems

Many psychotropic drugs, particularly major tranquilizers such as phenothiazines, may cause hepatic side-effects either by direct cytotoxicity or by inducing a cholestatic jaundice. The former mechanism usually becomes evident a short time after initiating therapy, while the latter may present early or late. Most commonly, liver enzyme changes are mild to moderate and do not require termination of therapy. Occasionally cholestatic jaundice will be severe and necessitate a change of drug. Also, occasionally, blood levels of other drugs requiring hepatic metabolism can be affected, though as often as not the clinician can make therapeutic (and economic) use of this. Screening liver tests initially or with continued therapy are not valuable unless the patient has pre-existing liver disease or a clinical problem.

Drugs which block histamine 2-receptors (e.g. tricyclics) may lower gastric acid secretion. While rarely a significant detriment, prolonged gastric acid suppression could in theory favor gastric malignancy, promote vitamin B12 deficiency or prevent the protective effect of stomach acid on invading ingested bacteria. Some other medications the absorption of which is influenced by gastric acidity could be affected. Occasionally this antihistamine-2 effect is useful and probably a patient treated with a tricyclic antidepressant would have no need to also take a conventional H-2 blocker as well. Anticholinergic psychotropics are very constipating. Elderly patients are at great risk because other factors, such as decreased activity, chronic low fluid intake, low bulk diet and the use of other constipating medications such as calcium channel blockers, are prevalent. Obstipation and impaction are frequent with potentially fatal results in the frail elderly. Impaction may be heralded only by delirium or behavioral change in the elderly who may have poor communication skills or low self-awareness. With chronic use, Ogilvie's syndrome or atonic megacolon may occur. Resection of the involved dilated colon only leads to further dilation of the remaining proximal bowel, or even the small bowel. A conservative approach is virtually always indicated.

Anticholinergic medications also decrease salivation. This frequently leads to an annoying dry mouth. Xerostomia may contribute to halitosis and malnutrition and occasionally becomes more significant if the effect combines with other factors leading to a decreased ability to swallow in a coordinated fashion. Choking, aspiration pneumonia or aspirated foreign body and asphyxia are possible. Antipsychotics, through dopamine antagonism, may affect the coordinated and complex process of swallowing and lead to dysphagia. Some patients will have visible difficulty in swallowing efficiently, others may fear aspiration and gradually or suddenly stop eating. This presentation may occur in the demented patient who is unable to communicate the swallowing problem to care givers, and so dysphagia from psychotropics (or other cause) should be considered in the geriatric patient who gradually or suddenly stops eating, or who stops eating a particular consistency of foods (solids, paste, liquid). Tardive dyskinesia may also decrease the ability to form a food bolus, present the bolus to the posterior pharynx in a coordinated fashion (in synchrony with respiratory effort), initiate and complete a swallow and/or clear the throat after swallowing.

Hematopoietic and lymphatic systems

Bone marrow function is potentially adversely affected by many psychotropic medications, particularly antipsychotics. Though risks of movement disorders are much reduced with clozapine, it is at the cost of much greater potential for leukopenia and even agranulocytosis. Risperidone seems to have the advantages of clozapine with respect to movement disorders, but retains relative safety in regard to hematopoiesis. Even high-potency butyrophenones have been implicated, however, and so probably all antipsychotics have potential for these effects. Leukopenia usually occurs soon after initiation of therapy, most often in two weeks to four months. Routine screening for this side-effect, however, is not worthwhile. Instead, at follow-up the physician should inquire about infections, fevers or pharyngitis and do a complete blood count only when history suggests a problem. Severe agranulocytosis from psychotropic medication can be fatal in up to one-third of cases. Though not approved by the United States Federal Drug Administration for this indication, this author has successfully treated clozapine-induced agranulocytosis with granulocyte colony-stimulating factor.

Lithium causes an increase in granulocytes in some cases. It is ineffective as a treatment for serious agranulocytosis, but can be used in cases of less serious leukopenia induced by antipsychotics when continued antipsychotic therapy is necessary. When used alone, lithium-induced leukocytosis with white counts twice or three times normal can be ignored.

Genitourinary system

A discussion of genitourinary side-effects of psychotropic drugs crosses the boundary with the endocrine system in the area of sexual dysfunction. These effects are described in the endocrine subsection of this chapter. Other genitourinary effects of psychotropic drugs, of course, are related to bladder function. The storage function of the bladder and the act of micturition are controlled in part by the central and peripheral nervous systems. Central tracts receive afferent messages from detrusor muscle stretch receptors via the spinal cord to the thalamus, reticular activating system, limbus, cerebellum and basal ganglia and into the detrusor reflex center located in the frontal lobe. The reader should note the several structures which share loci for emotionality and its expression. In the peripheral system, ganglia within the detrusor muscle connect with axons of the pelvic plexus and then on to the CNS. On the efferent side, tracts from lower sacral segments innervate the bladder wall and sphincter.

Parasympathetic stimulation (cholinergics) activates detrusor contraction and micturition while sympathetic stimulation (anticholinergic) is inhibitory. Thus, many anticholinergic drugs can induce urinary retention. In the elderly of either sex with detrusor instability and uninhibited bladder contractions caused by basal ganglia dysfunction (e.g. Alzheimer's disease and other neurodegenerative diseases), anticholinergic-induced urinary retention is particularly common. In males, prostatic hypertrophy may be additive. Patients may present with infrequent, incomplete or absent voiding and a palpable suprapubic mass. Also, the clinician should be alert to the paradoxical incontinence (overflow incontinence) which can occur with this side-effect.

Neurologic

Movement disorders

Movement disorders are relatively common side-effects in elders who receive antipsychotics and some other psychotropics. These may be of extrapyramidal (EPS) variety or tardive in nature. The EPS variety are generally quick to emerge after the onset of therapy and resolve when the offending agent is discontinued. The tardive type become apparent usually after long-term therapy and may resolve only very slightly or not at all when treatment is discontinued. EPS and tardive versions of drug-induced Parkinsonism, dyskinesia, dystonia, akathisia and myoclonus can occur. Elderly patients are at increased risk for EPS drug-induced Parkinsonian tremor, tardive dyskinesia and myoclonus, but at less risk for dystonia.

Drug-induced Parkinsonism may occur in one-quarter to more than one-half of elderly patients treated with conventional antipsychotics. Bradykinesia is the most prominent symptom and in conjunction with thermoregulatory dysfunction caused by antipsychotics, may lead to hypothermia. Other typical manifestations include expressionless face, cogwheel or lead-pipe rigidity, pill-rolling tremor, lack of conjugate arm swing, festination of the gait and a stooped forward-bending posture. This side-effect can be treated with anticholinergic drugs (e.g. benztropine, trihexyphenidyl, amantadine) which are usually discontinued after several months without re-exacerbation of the Parkinsonism. The anticholinergics, however, have their own risks in this age group (see anticholinergic side-effects) and if the Parkinsonism is sufficiently severe to warrant intervention, a switch to a non-conventional antipsychotic is reasonable.

Akathisia is defined by an extremely noxious feeling of inner restlessness. In the severely mentally ill or demented elder who lacks good communication skills, or when the treating physician fails to consider this possible side-effect, the syndrome can be mistakenly regarded as escalation of anxiety or psychosis. If so, the dose of the offending drug may be titrated upward with disastrous results. Little relief can be offered for the occasional unfortunate patient who goes unrecognized until the tardive variant of this movement disorder is established. The clinician should maintain considerable suspicion for this side-effect when upward titration of an antipsychotic has paradoxical effects on anxiety or agitated features.

Tardive dyskinesia can occur in some elders who have never been exposed to psychotropic drugs, characteristically emerging in some after dental work (e.g. new dentures). Most often it occurs after antipsychotic therapy. The risk is increased by the use of high-potency drugs, high doses and long-term use. Female sex and organic mental disorders also confer greater risk. Patients often display abnormal facial movements, e.g. lip smacking or pursing, sucking movements, tongue protrusion and chewing motions. Less often choreoathetoid movements of the head, neck and trunk can occur. These involuntary movements can be temporarily sublimated by the patient with effort, are worsened by anxiety and fatigue, are not present during sleep and in rare cases may be associated with perceptions of orofacial pain. Also, on rare occasions the muscles of respiration may be involved. The movements can be very socially disabling, and treatment is often ineffective or only partially helpful. An often unrecognized complication of tardive dyskinesia is the occurrence of swallowing disorders, a discussion of which occurs earlier in this chapter.

Atypical or non-neuroleptic antipsychotics have recently been developed which significantly reduce the risk of EPS movement disorders. Clozapine, followed by risperidone and olanzepine, have been marketed and several others are under investigation. Time will tell if these drugs also confer safety from tardive types of movement disorders, but early reports are very promising. Clozapine use is limited by blood dyscrasia while the safety from movement disorders of risperidone is limited to approved dosage. The non-neuroleptic antipsychotics also have enhanced effects on the negative symptoms of psychosis compared with ordinary antipsychotics.

Patients should give informed consent with documentation before receiving neuroleptic or other psychotropic drugs with the potential to cause tardive movement disorder. It is largely due to these potential side-effects that the prescription of psychotropic drugs in the USA is treated differently and more strictly in the law. In the interest of good care, patients receiving antipsychotic medications should be screened initially and periodically for movement disorders. Several scales exist for this purpose, such as the Abnormal Involuntary Movement Scale (AIMS) [7].

Seizures

Antipsychotics, cyclic antidepressants, selective serotonin uptake inhibitors and some other antidepressants lower seizure threshold and may induce seizures. The risk is not high with approximately 1% of the patients on antipsychotics experiencing seizures. Bupropion, among antidepressants, confers greater risk. An already impaired CNS, e.g. organic brain syndrome, prior history of epilepsy and alcohol abuse, will increase the risk. When psychotropic drugs of different classes are used in combination with each other, or with non-psychiatric drugs which also lower seizure threshold (e.g. caffeine, theophylline) the risk is compounded. Patients treated with these agents, and also receiving electroconvulsive therapy, have the advantage of lowered seizure threshold leading to longer and more intense seizures generated from lesser electrical stimuli. In theory, this should lead to better efficacy and fewer complications of electroconvulsive therapy (ECT).

Central anticholinergic syndrome

Up to one-third of elderly patients receiving a drug with anticholinergic effects may experience the central anticholinergic syndrome to some degree. Duplicate therapy (using multiple drugs with anticholinergic action) increases the risk. The syndrome is characterized by organic hallucinosis, agitated delirium and signs of parasympathetic stimulation, e.g. dilated pupils, blurred vision, dry mouth, flushed and dry skin, retention of urine and constipation. Cardiovascular effects include tachycardia, risk of arrhythmia and hypertension. Neurologic accompaniments include poor coordination, myoclonus or choreoathetosis. In milder cases the patient may exhibit paranoia, while in the extreme, an agitated delirium may progress to stupor and coma with hyperreflexia and signs of upper motor neuron dysfunction. The condition can be fatal, especially in elderly patients with significant co-morbidity such as cardiovascular disease.

Neuroleptic malignant syndrome

Antipsychotic medications may rarely cause a syndrome of hyperpyrexia, rhabdomyolysis with rigidity, extrapyramidal symptoms and coma called neuroleptic malignant syndrome (NMS). The etiology of this disorder is unknown but it is related to dopamine antagonism and no consistent predictive risk factors exist. This serious and potentially fatal adverse event occurs early in treatment with an antipsychotic. In the past, it was believed that the elderly had a lower risk than younger patients, but more recent studies indicate that this was an artifact of underrecognition in the geriatric population in whom agitation, rigidity, autonomic instability and delirium or coma are more easily blamed on other conditions. NMS may be treated with supportive measures, especially anticipating renal failure. Drug therapy is controversial but dantrolene sodium, bromocriptine and amantadine have been used. The former has proven most effective.

Oddly, the condition is not specific to a particular neuroleptic, nor is rechallenge with the offending agent necessarily contraindicated once NMS is successfully resolved, though few practitioners have the intestinal fortitude to resume such a treatment after so serious an episode. NMS may be confused with serotonin syndrome, a description of which follows along with a discussion of the differential diagnosis.

Serotonin syndrome

A syndrome of serotonin hyperstimulation has been reported as the result of exposure to psychotropics which have effects on this neurotransmitter. Most often case reports involve combination therapy of a selective serotonin reuptake inhibitor or clomipramine (a tricyclic which has fairly unique serotonin-blocking properties), along with a drug favoring serotonin production (tryptophan, theophylline) or a drug slowing serotonin degradation (MAOIs). Frequently, cases occur due not to intended combination therapy, but as the result of too rapid switching of one agent to another and not allowing a 'washout' of five times the half-life of the discontinued drug (Chapter 2). Patients with serotonin syndrome have an altered mental state, behavioral symptoms, altered muscle tone and autonomic instability. Agitation, delirium, incoordination, coma and seizure may occur, with delirium being most common. Myoclonus is the second most frequent feature with rigidity, hyperreflexia, tremor and shivering also seen. Patients typically may be either hypertensive or hypotensive, but consistently have tachycardia, hyperpyrexia and diaphoresis. Withdrawal of the offending agent(s) and supportive management are required treatments. Myoclonus has been reported to respond to cyproheptadine therapy.

Hyperpyrexia, diaphoresis, rhabdomyolysis, followed by possible disseminated intravascular coagulation and acute renal failure, are symptoms shared by both the serotonin syndrome and neuroleptic malignant syndrome. Both are potentially fatal iatrogenic diseases making a differential diagnosis and a specific treatment critically important for the patient and physician alike. For those patients on neuroleptics and SSRIs (a not unlikely clinical circumstance) this constellation of symptoms creates a very difficult diagnostic dilemma. In serotonin syndrome the agitation and hyperreflexia are more likely to be exaggerated symptoms and myoclonus is nearly always present. In NMS a more impressive autonomic dysfunction and rigidity should help clarify the diagnosis. Finally, a history of too rapid a change in drugs affecting the serotonin systems or combination therapy should be present.

The serotonin syndrome serves as an important reminder of therapeutic axioms encouraging clinicians to 'start low and go slow', to avoid polypharmacy and to avoid treating symptoms rather than disease states.

Dependence and addiction

Benzodiazepines and methylphenidate (frequently used in geropsychiatry) together with amphetamines, barbiturates and methylquinolone, and meprobamate (less frequently used) have the potential for causing physical dependence and therefore addiction. A drug with the ability to cause dependence will cause withdrawal symptoms when discontinued. In some individuals treated with such a drug, the rewards of drug effect and/or the need to avoid withdrawal symptoms leads to addiction defined by drug-seeking behavior. Special characteristics of drugs make them potentially more likely to cause dependence and addiction. Tolerance or tachyphylaxis is the pharmacologic characteristic for repeated doses of a drug to cause less and less effect. A corollary is that with increasing tolerance, a particular dose will eventually not ward off withdrawal symptoms. Drugs with more immediate and appreciable activity and with shorter half-lives are more prone to lead to addiction (the cocktail effect).

Often withdrawal effects are very similar to the psychiatric symptoms being treated in the first place. Benzodiazepines, barbiturates, methaquinolone and meprobamate used for sedation or sleep will cause rebound insomnia on withdrawal. Benzodiazepines used as anxiolytics may cause agitation on withdrawal. Methylphenidate may cause depression when stopped suddenly. In such cases the clinician will have difficulty in determining whether the problem on termination of therapy is a relapse or withdrawal symptoms. Patients almost invariably view the discomfort as a relapse and demand continuation of the addicting drug. Psychological addiction (without potential for physical withdrawal) can occur with virtually any psychotropic or non-psychotropic drug in the elderly patient, especially when the medication or the illness behavior for which it is prescribed fills a 'special need' in the patient's life. The use of many physically addictive drugs is probably also supported by these same psychological factors.

The clinician should consider addiction potential before choosing among the potentially addicting and non-addicting therapeutic possibilities. A prior history of substance abuse such as alcohol, tobacco, obsessive/compulsive traits or bipolar illness are relative contraindications to highly addictive drugs.

In some cases therapeutic withdrawal is essential to the eventual success of treatment. For instance, gradual termination of a misused benzodiazepine may be required before a resistant major depression will improve. A switch to an ultralong-acting benzodiazepine, such as clorazepate, given on a scheduled basis, not *pro re nata*, and then gradually tapered over many months can be safe and successful. Rapid termination, especially in the very old and infirm, is cruel and could even be fatal. In many cases where therapeutic goals are limited, the physician may choose to control the addiction rather than aspiring to correct it.

Psychobehavioral effects

Good research into the psychomotor and psychobehavioral effects of psychotropic medication is confounded by many factors: premorbid personality, affective state, the effect of practice and learning on repeated trials are examples. It seems certain that psychoactive drugs have the potential to affect simple and complex psychomotor functioning adversely. This may lead to decreased functional ability and may even decrease socialization, especially if sedation is involved. On the other hand, the therapeutic effect on pathology may outweigh the negative psychomotor effects on performance in socialization. For example, even though a benzodiazepine may be causing some sedation in an elder with generalized anxiety disorder, the positive effects on attention span may lead to better performance or better social interactions. The clinician must consistently weigh risks and benefits.

Falls

Barbiturates, antidepressants, major tranquilizers and long-acting benzo-diazepines have all been associated with increased falls in the elderly. Sedation, postural hypotension and possibly negative psychomotor effects on reaction time and perceptual ability and judgment are mechanisms. Elders already suffer a decline in proprioception, various physiologic changes increasing their susceptibility to postural hypotension and often have lower limb dysfunction, neurologic or sensory deficits. To compound the elderly's risk of injury with falls, osteoarthritis and osteoporosis, stiffness and weakness from disuse, and senile atrophy of the skin are prevalent. Falling begets fear and lowered self-esteem, and a vicious cycle of involutional behavior with atrophy as a consequence of decreased activity. Falling is a significant predictor of physical decline and death in the elderly.

The increased risk of hip fracture from several psychotropic classes in a long-term care population has been studied by Ray *et al.* [8].

Emotional changes

Psychotropic drugs may cause emotional changes other than the expected therapeutic ones. In this author's experience, this is most often the case in patients with organic impairments. Buspirone may increase anxiety and problem behavior in some patients. SSRIs fairly frequently cause anxiety. There is weaker evidence to implicate them as the cause of impulsive and aggressive acts, though several persons in the USA have used a 'Prozac made me do it' defense for criminal behavior. Any sedative drug may cause anxiety, agitation or heightened suspiciousness in a patient with paranoia who abhors the sense of lost control or alertness.

Opinions are mixed in the literature regarding beta-blocker induced depression, but newer studies assert this side-effect does not occur. In theory, water-soluble beta-blockers should be safer than lipid-soluble ones as they would have less ability to cross the blood–brain barrier. However, if the beta-blocker is used as a psychotherapeutic agent (e.g. treatment of aggression in an organically impaired patient and of anxiety in the UK), the physician must choose a lipid-soluble drug for the same reason. Similarly, benzodiazepines have long been implicated in drug-induced depression, but careful review finds this is not so. Reserpine, once used as an antipsychotic and now occasionally used for treatment of hypertension or tardive dyskinesia, does cause depression in some persons.

Suicidality

Increased suicidal ideation and behavior have been linked by clinical observation to several classes of psychotropic medication and specifically to maprotiline, diazepam, amitriptyline and fluoxetine. Controlled clinical trials have not clearly supported concerns that these occurrences are mediated by specific neurochemical effects on suicidal ideation. An increased incidence of suicide in the early phases of treatment may also be explained by a 'roll back phenomenon', which theorizes the depressed patient must emerge from depression by back-tracking through the stages of their disease. A related theory suggests that energizing a suicidal patient who is too severely psychomotor retarded to create or act on a suicidal plan will put the patient in jeopardy as they begin to 'improve'. Others have suggested that when a treatment is started but is not yet effective, or the patient returns to their home environment after visiting the therapist only to find things are just as they were before, a renewed sense of hopelessness may cause a suicidal act.

Still, neurochemical deficiencies have been found in patients who attempt or complete suicide. Homovanillic acid (HVA), precursor of dopamine, and 5-hydroxy indoleacetic acid(5-HIAA), precursor of serotonin, have been found to be deficient in these patients. Fluoxetine, in particular, was the target of much concern as a drug which could induce suicidality. Scant evidence exists that fluoxetine in the early stages would downregulate serotonin systems before having its known effect of enhancement. It is possible that stimulating one monoamine may cause a compensatory depletion of another. A surge of serotonin, induced by fluoxetine (or other SSRI), could in theory downregulate dopamine and lead to a tardive akathisia. Patients may become so distressed with akathisia as to become suicidal.

The clinician should remain aware that antidepressants are highly pharmacoactive agents with relatively narrow therapeutic to toxic ratios. SSRIs and other classes are relatively safer than tricyclics, mostly as a result of decreased cardiotoxicity. Specifically, the tricyclic antidepressants qualify as almost perfect poisons because we give these drugs, of necessity, to patients at great risk of making suicide attempts. There is difficulty in monitoring to see if the patient is hoarding enough medicine to take an overdose, even if we prescribe only small, safe amounts. There is no good antidote for toxicity with these agents, nor can they be cleared by dialysis.

SUMMARY

The side-effects of psychotropic drugs in the elderly are myriad. They may be difficult to recognize even in a patient whose clinical course is devastated by adverse drug reactions. Only a good working knowledge of the pharmacology and pharmacodynamics of the drugs we prescribe and a constant vigilance will prevent us from breaking the command-ment *'primum non nocere'*, first do no harm. Vigilance implies not only sus-picion, self-awareness and humility, but also an objective scientific approach to an area of medicine that has in the past been quite subjec-tive. A working diagnosis and a degree of confidence in that diagnosis must be determined. Psychotropic drugs are chosen as treatments for dis-eases, not for symptoms [9]. Various instruments should be employed to objectively assess the functional, cognitive, behavioral and emotional sta-tus of the patient at baseline and periodically during therapy. Target symptoms and therapeutic goals, plans for the duration of therapy and the place of pharmacotherapy within a total treatment plan should be established *before* the drugs are initiated. Once drugs are prescribed, methods and time tables for monitoring efficacy and common or serious side-effects should be established. Finally, when an elderly patient changes status for the worse, the medication regimen must always be reviewed with a drug reaction in mind.

REFERENCES

1. Smith, D.A. (1995) *Geriatric Psychopathology: Delivering Quality Care to Nursing Home Residents: OBRA Regulations and Beyond.* Behavioral Health Resource Press, Providence, Rhode Island, USA.
2. Beers, M., Avorn, J., Soumerai, S.B. *et al.* (1988) Psychoactive medication use in intermediate-care facility residents. *JAMA* **260**, 3016.
3. Federal Register. (1989) Requirements for long-term care facilities. *Fed. Register* **54** (249), 53611–53612.
4. Federal Register. (1992) Proposed changes to the long-term care facility (SNF and NF) requirements. *Fed. Register* **57**, 4517.
5. Stoudemire, A. and Smith, D.A. (1996) OBRA regulations and the use of psy-chotropic drugs in long-term care facilities: impact and implication for geropsychiatric care. *Gen. Hosp. Psychiatry* **18**, 77.
6. Sloane, P. and Lekan-Rutledge, D. (1988) Drug prescribing by telephone: a potential cause of polypharmacy in nursing homes. *JAGS* **36**, 574.
7. Rockville, G.W. (ed.) (1976) National Institute of Mental Health: Abnormal Involuntary Movement Scale. In *ECDEV Assessment Manual.* National Institute of Mental Health, USA.
8. Ray, W.A., Griffin, M.R., Schaffner, W. *et al.* (1987) Psychotropic drug use and the risk of hip fracture. *N. Engl. J. Med.* **316**, 363.
9. Hall, R.C.W. (1980) *Psychiatric Presentations of Medical Illness: Somatopsychic Disorders.* SD Medical and Scientific Books, New York, USA.

Part Two

Cognitive disorders

4

Neurochemical substrates of dementia

Julian Gray and Albert Enz

INTRODUCTION

The development of levodopa for the treatment of Parkinson's disease was a success story for the neurochemical approach to drug development for a neurological disorder: a neurotransmitter deficit was found and a replacement therapy developed. More recently, based on the deficits in cholinergic neurotransmission observed in Alzheimer brain, symptomatic therapies with cholinergic drugs have been developed (see below and Chapter 6), with clinical benefit at least in a proportion of patients.

A justifiable objection to the neurochemical approach to understanding the dementias is that it avoids addressing the fundamental underlying pathophysiological problems of the disease. Nevertheless, increasing evidence suggests that neurochemical changes may play a role not only in the evolution of symptoms, but also in certain pathological processes, such as amyloid misprocessing or free radical production, as discussed below. A better understanding of the neurochemical substrates of dementia could therefore help in designing not only symptomatic but even disease-modifying approaches to treatment.

In this chapter we summarise some of the main changes observed in the commonest cause of dementia, Alzheimer's disease. A brief discussion is then made of the less advanced state of knowledge concerning the neurochemical substrates of some of the rarer dementias that affect the elderly.

Psychopharmacology of Cognitive and Psychiatric Disorders in the Elderly. Edited by David Wheatley and David Smith. Published in 1998 by Chapman and Hall, London. ISBN 0 412 82470 1

ALZHEIMER'S DISEASE

Most of the work on neurochemical changes in Alzheimer's disease is derived from observations on post-mortem tissue, with the exception of isolated studies of brain biopsy material. In spite of reservations concerning the reliability and specificity of changes seen in post-mortem tissue, certain neurochemical changes appear consistently as summarised in Table 4.1.

The cholinergic deficit

The best documented neurochemical change in Alzheimer's disease is the cholinergic deficit resulting from degeneration of cholinergic neurons, especially in the neocortex and hippocampus [1]. Biochemically, the loss of cholinergic neurons is mirrored by:

- reduced activity of choline acetyltransferase (ChAT), the enzyme involved in the synthesis of acetylcholine
- reduced activity of acetylcholinesterase (AChE), the enzyme which metabolises acetylcholine
- reduced activity of the reuptake system for choline, the precursor of acetylcholine.

Acetylcholine receptors are also affected by the disease process. Although the postsynaptic muscarinic receptors (m_1 subtype) have been found to be intact, a loss of presynaptic muscarinic receptors (m_2 subtype)

Table 4.1 Neurochemical changes that appear consistently in Alzheimer's disease

System	Transmitter level	Receptors	
Acetylcholine	↓	M1→	M2↓
Monoamines			
Noradrenaline	↓	α→	β→
Dopamine	→(↓)	D1↓	D2→
Serotonin	↓	S1↓	S2↓
Amino acids			
GABA	→(↓)	→	
Glutamate	→(↓)	↓	
Peptides			
SRIF	↓	↓	
CRF	↓	↑	
Substance P	→	↓	

↓: decrease; ↑: increase; →: unchanged;
CRF: Corticotrophin-releasing factor; SRIF: somatostatin reactive immune factor

has been reported. Nicotinic receptors, the other main receptors for acetylcholine, are also reduced in number. Interestingly, nicotine itself has been shown to produce some positive cognitive effects in Alzheimer patients [2]. The loss of cholinergic neurons is observed not only in the cortex but also in subcortical neuronal systems, especially the **ascending cholinergic neurons** which arise from the basal nucleus of Meynert in the basal forebrain and project to the cortex (Fig. 4.1).

Is the cholinergic deficit related to the symptoms in Alzheimer's disease?

There is now strong evidence that some of the symptoms of Alzheimer's disease are related to the cholinergic deficits described above. This conclusion rests on three observations:

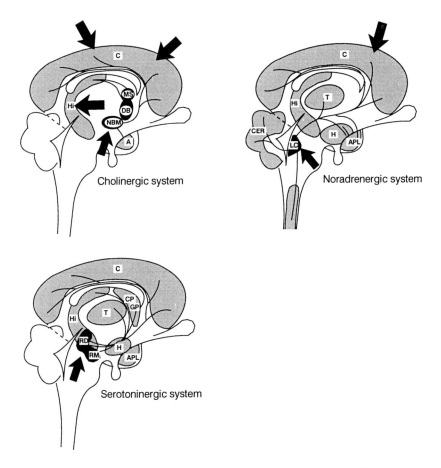

Fig. 4.1 Monoamine pathways that may be involved in Alzheimer's disease.

1. The loss of cholinergic markers in the brains of patients at post-mortem has been shown in some studies to be correlated with the degree of dementia and with the number of plaques [3].
2. Anticholinergic drugs such as scopolamine have been shown to impair learning and memory in animals and humans. Similarly, lesions of the ascending cholinergic tracts in animals lead to cognitive dysfunction which may be reversed by cholinergic drugs.
3. Cholinergic drugs such as the acetylcholinesterase inhibitors have been shown to improve cognitive function in a proportion of patients with mild to moderate dementia of the Alzheimer type (Chapter 6).

Recently, the possibility has been raised that hypofunction of cholinergic neurons could be involved in the pathogenesis of the altered metabolism of amyloid proteins observed in Alzheimer's disease (Chapter 5). This hypothesis stems from the finding that the processing and secretion of amyloid precursor protein (APP) is influenced by muscarinic (m_1) receptors [4]. The question as to whether long-term treatment with cholinergic drugs could influence disease progression, through interaction with amyloid metabolism, must be answered by long-term controlled clinical trials.

Monoamines

The cholinergic system is by no means the only one affected in Alzheimer's disease. There is also good evidence for a loss of monoaminergic neurons, including the ascending pathways for noradrenaline and serotonin analogous to those for the cholinergic neurons (Fig. 4.1).

Reduced noradrenergic neurotransmission

This is reflected by a reduction in activity of dopamine beta-hydroxylase, the enzyme responsible for the synthesis of noradrenaline. Losses of noradrenergic neurons are seen especially in the locus ceruleus of the midbrain and cortex [5]. There is some evidence for a compensatory increase in metabolism of noradrenaline in the affected brain regions.

Reduced serotoninergic (5-HT) neurotransmission

Similar evidence for this is found in post-mortem studies. Decreased concentrations of serotonin have been measured in the temporal cortex, hippocampus and basal ganglia at post-mortem, while even more pronounced reductions in serotonin concentration were observed in cortical biopsy samples taken in patients about 3.5 years after the onset of dementia [6]. There is also evidence for reduced numbers of 5-HT_1 and 5-HT_2 receptors in the cortex and hippocampus.

Dopaminergic neurotransmission

Overall there is little evidence for a significant alteration in **dopaminergic neurotransmission** in Alzheimer's disease.

Are the monoaminergic deficits related to the symptoms of Alzheimer's disease?

The link between the monoaminergic deficit and symptoms of Alzheimer's disease is less well understood than that of the cholinergic deficit. Nevertheless, certain observations do suggest such a link. There is good evidence from animal experiments that both noradrenergic and serotoninergic neurons play a role in the processes of learning and memory. The noradrenergic systems have been particularly implicated in the processes of arousal, attention and concentration, while many studies show important involvement of serotoninergic neurons in the regulation of mood, sleep and appetite behaviors which are very often disrupted in Alzheimer patients. Deciding how important such neurochemical lesions are in individual patients in contributing to cognitive and behavioral disturbances is very difficult. Few studies of highly selective agents for noradrenaline or serotonin receptors have been published. Studies with selective serotonin reuptake inhibitors have not shown dramatic effects, but indicate that improvements in mood may occur especially in patients with concomitant depression [7]. Improvements in cognitive function have been observed after selegiline, an inhibitor of monoamine oxidase B (MAO-B) [8]. Theoretically, the amphetamine-like effects of selegiline could play a role in its actions, so that results of studies with drugs more specific in their actions must be awaited before it can be concluded that the symptomatic effects are due to MAO-B inhibition.

The possibility has also been raised recently that inhibition of MAO-B could influence disease progression. An increase in the activity of MAO-B has been consistently demonstrated in Alzheimer cortex at postmortem, and has been localised especially to astrocytes surrounding senile plaques [9]. MAO-B is involved in the deamination of dopamine and trace amines such as phenylethylamine. During this deamination, hydrogen peroxide is formed which, through a reaction with iron, leads to the generation of hydroxy radicals. These free radicals are highly toxic to neurons and can also promote the aggregation of soluble amyloid into insoluble forms. An increase in MAO-B activity could therefore increase the formation of free radicals, leading to oxidative stress and the increased deposition of amyloid. Assessment of the clinical relevance of these changes must await the results of long-term studies with MAO-B inhibitors such as selegiline and more selective agents such as lazabemide (Chapter 6).

Amino acids

The amino acid glutamate is now recognised to have a pivotal role as a neurotransmitter for rapid signalling, in addition to its role in normal metabolism. There is evidence that glutamate is a principal neurotransmitter of the corticocortical association fibres and the hippocampal pathways, which degenerate early in Alzheimer's disease [10]. Studies on the levels of glutamate and its receptors have overall confirmed the predicted reductions. The situation is less clear for GABA, the major inhibitory amino acid neurotransmitter. Overall there is no evidence for major changes in its neurochemical pathology in Alzheimer's disease.

Neuropeptides

There is animal evidence for a role for several neuropeptides in learning and memory, including (among others) somatostatin, corticotrophin-releasing factor (CRF), vasopressin and neuropeptide Y [10]. While various studies have shown regional reductions in their activity in Alzheimer's disease, the relation between these findings and the clinical symptomatology in Alzheimer's disease patients remains unclear. Clinical studies with vasopressin and somatostatin analogues have failed to show clearcut clinical effects, though these results have to be interpreted with caution in view of the uncertain blood–brain barrier penetration of such agents.

Multiple neurotransmitter deficits as an important substrate for dementia

It is clear from the above discussion that any attempt to understand the neurochemical substrates of Alzheimer's disease must acknowledge that the symptoms are likely to result from disturbances in several interacting neurotransmitter systems.

Animal studies have shown that the integrity of the noradrenergic pathways may be important to the effective functioning of the ascending cholinergic neurons in cognition. A combined lesion of these pathways, as seen in Alzheimer's disease, could therefore have particularly profound effects. Future treatment strategies are likely to see more attempts at multiple neurotransmitter replacement, in spite of the attendant methodological complexity. Encouragement for this approach comes from a pilot study combining the acetylcholinesterase inhibitor physostigmine with the MAO-B inhibitor selegiline, in which additive effects on cognition were observed [11].

OTHER DEMENTIAS

Multi-infarct and mixed dementias

Multi-infarct and 'mixed' (Alzheimer's type with vascular) dementias are common (constituting up to 20% each of the total number of dementia cases). The finding of vascular changes in the brains of many Alzheimer's disease cases is anyway not surprising in view of the widespread vascular deposition of amyloid [12]. Systemic studies of the neurochemistry of vascular and mixed Alzheimer's disease/vascular dementias are lacking at present.

Pick's disease

In Pick's disease, cerebral atrophy is usually confined to the frontal and temporal regions, with some associated gliosis and 'Pick bodies' seen in the neurons. Senile plaques are infrequent and neurofibrillary tangles absent. Although reduction of neurons in the nucleus basalis of Meynert has been reported, loss of cholinergic markers in the cortex does not occur, in contrast to Alzheimer's disease.

Lewy body disease

F.H. Lewy described eosinophilic inclusions in neurons in the human brain which are called Lewy bodies [13], occurring in a range of neuro-degenerative diseases. Diffuse Lewy body disease is an important cause of dementia and is characterised by widespread deposition of Lewy bodies in the cerebral cortex and subcortical sites. The clinical picture features prominent early psychiatric symptoms including hallucinations. Neurochemically, a marked cortical cholinergic deficit has been reported [14]. Of interest in this regard was the finding that patients responding to the acetylcholinesterase inhibitor tacrine in a clinical study were subsequently shown to have Lewy body disease at post-mortem [14,15].

Subcortical dementias

In the subcortical dementias cell loss occurs in deep grey matter rather than in the cerebral cortex. Subcortical dementia is most frequently observed in degenerative disease associated with basal ganglia lesions and movement disorders, notably Parkinson's disease, Huntington's chorea and progressive supranuclear palsy.

Parkinson's disease

Up to 30% of patients with Parkinson's disease have some degree of dementia [16]. The aetiology is complex, as a proportion of patients also have the pathological features of Alzheimer's disease in the cortex. There is evidence that, independent of any coexisting Alzheimer-type pathology, dementia in Parkinsonian patients may occur due to lesions of important subcortical neuronal systems, and subcorticocortical pathways. The major lesions identified to date include the following.

Nigrostriatal dopaminergic pathway

This, the classic dopaminergic lesion of Parkinson's disease, may also be implicated in the pathogenesis of intellectual deterioration. This may be due to impairment in related output pathways to the cerebral cortex, such as the nigrothalamocortical pathway and the striato-pallido-thalamocortical pathway.

Mesocorticolimbic dopaminergic pathway

Evidence suggests that mesocortical and mesolimbic dopaminergic pathways degenerate in Parkinson's disease, and that this loss is greater in demented patients.

Ceruleocortical pathway

The pathway from the locus ceruleus to the cerebral cortex degenerates with loss of its neurotransmitter noradrenaline, especially in the amygdala, hippocampus and frontal cortex. Animal studies suggest that such a lesion may be associated with deficits in attention, learning and memory.

Raphe-cortical serotoninergic neurons

Ascending serotoninergic neurons are partially lesioned in Parkinsonian patients, leading to reductions in serotonin concentrations especially in the hippocampus, frontal cortex, cingular and entorhinal cortex. In view of the known role for serotonin in learning and affect, it is likely that the serotonergic deficiency plays a role in Parkinsonian dementia.

Ascending cholinergic pathways

Loss of ascending cholinergic neuronal pathways has also been detected in Parkinsonian patients and linked with impairment of acetylcholine-dependent cognitive function.

Huntington's disease

In addition to chorea, mood disturbances, psychosis and subcortical dementia also occur in this disease. There is progressive loss of spiny neurons in the corpus striatum, with associated gliosis. Subsequent pathological abnormalities occur in the globus pallidus, thalamus, sub-thalamic nucleus, brain stem and spinal cord.

The neurochemical substrate of the dementia is mixed: the most marked biochemical change is a 50–90% reduction in gamma-amino-butyric acid in the striatum [17]. The cholinergic system is generally spared in contrast to the situation in Alzheimer's disease. Other biochem-ical abnormalities include reductions in the density of substance P and metenkephalin, and an increase in somatostatin levels in the striatum. The degree to which the neuropeptide alterations are linked to the dementia is not clear.

CONCLUSION

The recent positive results with cholinergic therapy such as tacrine and the newer acetylcholinesterase inhibitors in Alzheimer's disease have highlighted the importance of understanding the neurochemical sub-strates of the disease in devising improved treatments. The role of non-cholinergic neurotransmitter changes in the dementia is not proven, but alterations in noradrenaline and serotonin function are likely to con-tribute to the evolution of the cognitive, affective and behavioral distur-bances seen. So far, it is hard to gauge the clinical importance of alterations in neuropeptide levels and function. It is likely that multiple transmitter disturbances combine to produce the final clinical picture, and that multiple neurotransmitter treatments would be more effective than monotherapy affecting only one neurochemical system. This remains to be tested in practice and will be a challenge for clinical researchers. More research is needed to better understand the neuro-chemical substrates of non-Alzheimer dementias. The value of such research may be enhanced by the possibility that neurochemical changes may be linked not only to symptomatology, but also to underlying patho-logical events, such as the recently discovered link between acetylcholine and amyloid processing.

REFERENCES

1. Perry, E.K., Marshall, E., Kerwin, J. *et al.* (1986) The cholinergic hypothesis: ten years on. *Br. Med. Bull.* **42**, 63–69.
2. Sahakian, B., Jones, G., Levy, R. *et al.* (1989) The effects of nicotine on atten-tion, information processing and short-term memory in patients with dementia of the Alzheimer type. *Br. J. Psychiatry* **154**, 797–800.

3. Perry, E.K., Tomlinson, B.E., Blessed, G. *et al.* (1978) Correlation of cholinergic abnormalities with senile plaques and mental test scores in senile dementia. *Br. Med. J.* **2**, 1457–1459.

4. Nitsch, R.M., Slack, B.E., Wurtman, R.J. and Growdon, J.H. (1992) Release of Alzheimer amyloid precursor derivatives stimulated by activation of muscarinic acetylcholine receptors. *Science* **258**, 304–307.

5. Tomlinson, B.E., Irving, D. and Blessed, G. (1981) Cell loss in the locus coeruleus in senile dementia of the Alzheimer type. *J. Neurol. Sci.* **49**, 418–421.

6. Palmer, A.M., Frances, P.T., Benton, J.S. *et al.* (1987) Catecholaminergic neurons assessed antemortem in Alzheimer's disease. *Brain Res.* **414**, 365–375.

7. Gottfries, C.G. (1994) Therapy options in Alzheimer's disease. *Br. J. Clin. Pract.* **48**, 327–330.

8. Tariot, P.N., Cohen, R.M. and Sunderland, T. (1987) L-deprenyl in Alzheimer's disease. *Arch. Gen. Psychiatry* **44**, 427–433.

9. Saura, J., Luque, J.M., Cesura, A.M. *et al.* (1994) Increased monoamine oxidase B activity in plaque-associated astrocytes of Alzheimer brains revealed by quantitative enzyme radioautography. *Neuroscience* **62**, 15–30.

10. Francis, P.T., Cross, A.J. and Bowen, D.M. (1994) Neurotransmitters and neuropeptides. In *Alzheimer's Disease*, eds Terry, R.D., Katzman, R. and Blick, K.L, pp. 247–261, Raven Press, New York.

11. Schneider, L.S., Olin, J.T. and Pawluczyk, S. (1993) A double-blind crossover pilot study of L-deprenyl (selegiline) combined with cholinesterase inhibitor in Alzheimer's disease. *Am. J. Psychiatry* **150**, 321–323.

12. Ellis, R.J., Olichney, J.M., Thal, L.J. *et al.* (1996) Cerebral amyloid angiopathy in the brains of patients with Alzheimer's disease: the CERAD experience, part XV. *Neurology* **46**, 1592–1596.

13. Gibb, W.R.G. and Poewe, V.H. (1986) The centenary of Friedrich H. Lewy. *Neuropathol. Appl. Neurobiol.* **12**, 217–221.

14. Liberini, P., Valerio, A., Memo, M. and Spano, P. (1996) Lewy-body dementia and responsiveness to cholinesterase inhibitors: a paradigm for heterogeneity of Alzheimer's disease? *Trends Pharmacol. Sci.* **17**, 155–160.

15. Levy, R. (1994) Lewy bodies and response to tacrine in Alzheimer's disease. *Lancet* **343**, 176.

16. Agid, Y., Ruberg, M., Dubois, B. and Javoy-Agid., F. (1984) Biochemical substrates of mental disturbance in Parkinson's disease. In *Advances in Neurology*, vol. 40, *Parkinson-specific Motor and Mental Disorders*, eds Hassler, R.G. and Christ, J.F., pp. 211–218. Raven Press, New York.

17. Perry, T.L., Hansen, S. and Kloster, M. (1973) Huntington's disease: deficiency of aminobutyric acid in brain. *N. Engl. J. Med.* **288**, 337–342.

5

Neuropathological implications for therapy

Danielle Fallin, Nancy Tresser and Michael Mullan

INTRODUCTION

Neuropathology has been the cornerstone of diagnosis and research in the senile dementias for several decades. Much of the focus of research has resulted from primary observations of the pathology of these disorders. Neurochemistry, immunohistochemistry, *in situ* RNA analysis, DNA analysis and other techniques have added key pieces to the description and the understanding of many of these disorders. Logically, neuropathological implications for therapy should be derived from observations that reflect the etiology of a disorder. The major shortcoming of neuropathological data in the consideration of etiology is the absence of an accurate temporal dimension. The exact onset of disease pathology and rate of progression are difficult to accurately quantify clinically and impossible to follow pathologically except in those rare cases of brain biopsy. Although neuropathology has provided the backbone for the analysis of all the dementias and gives the best clues to etiology in the acute onset dementias such as the infarct dementias, it is less helpful in the chronic insidious onset disorders. In these disorders the question always arises as to whether the observed neuropathology is a cause or a consequence of the disease.

This type of question is crucial to the development of a rational drug therapy. In no other disorder is this issue more problematic than in

Psychopharmacology of Cognitive and Psychiatric Disorders in the Elderly. Edited by David Wheatley and David Smith. Published in 1998 by Chapman and Hall, London. ISBN 0 412 82470 1

Alzheimer's disease. In this disorder there is an ongoing controversy over whether amyloid deposition is a result of the disease process or whether it is responsible for neuronal loss. Similar questions apply to the pathology seen in the other primary degenerative disorders. Molecular genetic errors linked to a disorder provide two important ways to explore issues of etiology. Firstly, genetic mutations become the first step in theoretical pathogenic pathways. Secondly, they provide the substrate for molecular modeling of the disease in cell culture or more completely in transgenic animals. It is hoped, for instance, that the production of transgenic animals containing genetic errors known to trigger the disease in humans will allow accurate animal modeling. Features of such animals that are regarded as evidence that the disease process has been successfully mimicked are widely taken to be neuropathological rather than behavioral or cognitive. Thus in Alzheimer's disease deposition of amyloid is regarded as an essential feature of accurate transgenic animal models of the disease. Transgenic animals offer the ability to sequentially analyze the pathological changes triggered by mutant human genes. The relation of pathology to cognitive impairment and of the effects of therapy can be similarly established in such animals. Recent advances in the transgenic animal modeling of Alzheimer's disease [1] ensure that future chapters on the topic of neuropathological implications for treatment will include data on the effects of known and new therapies on the Alzheimer's neuropathology in these animals. It is anticipated that such modeling will expedite drug discovery in Alzheimer's and other dementias by removing the requirement for detailed understanding of disease processes before drug testing can begin.

Aside from empirical applications of the molecular genetic discoveries in Alzheimer's disease, their advent has resulted in coherent, if unproven, molecular theories of etiology. Consequently therapies based on these discoveries are already emerging. In addition, pharmacotherapies based on more classic analyses of Alzheimer's are currently available and in experimental stages. In addition to the specific discoveries associated with particular dementias, other theories drive the therapeutic discovery process. For instance, the free radical theory of aging is broadly applied to the development of antioxidants in a wide range of neurodegenerative disorders. The absence of specific details of free radical imbalance in most cases currently inhibits the development of correspondingly specific pharmacotherapy. Of the primary neurodegenerative dementias Alzheimer's is given the greatest attention in this chapter because it is the commonest dementia and consequently is receiving most of the focus of drug development for dementia in the elderly. Vascular dementia, a group of disorders, some of which are poorly understood, are also receiving much pharmacological attention, either directly or in relation to their underlying disorders such as cardiac disease or hypertension.

ALZHEIMER'S DISEASE

Introduction

Alzheimer's disease (AD) is a common dementing mental disorder among the older populations of developed countries. It is characterized clinically by an insidious global loss of cognitive functioning and pathologically by cortical deposition of β amyloid plaques and the development of neurofibrillary tangles (NFTs) as well as neuronal death. This debilitating disease affects a few percent of the population over 65 years, but unfortunately shows an exponential increase in incidence and prevalence with age. It is the third leading cause of death in the USA behind heart disease and cancer, and is the leading cause of institutionalization. The relentless progression and extended disease course exact both a psychological and economic toll on the spouse or major caregiver. At end-stage AD the affected individual is generally relegated to full-time medical treatment. It has been estimated that the annual cost incurred for one AD patient is around $47 000, which amounts to around $67 billion for society overall [2]. With this economic and emotional burden it is clear that even a small improvement in treatment or prevention could result in large benefits and savings. The present goals of therapy therefore are mostly aimed at shifting the exponential incidence curve to the right so that for a given population the age of onset is delayed and/or the rate of progression is decreased.

Clinical description and diagnosis

The hallmark clinical feature of AD is the gradual, insidious onset of memory loss, beginning with most recently learned information and progressing to loss of the most overlearnt knowledge. This disease is often subgrouped on the basis of age at disease onset with an age border of 65 years arbitrarily segregating late and early onset groups. Although the two groups are virtually identical clinically, this differentiation correlates with etiologic heterogeneity, early onset familial cases being caused by genetic mutations, late onset cases having a complex, multifactorial etiology. The disease progresses steadily, eventually resulting in death around 7 years after onset, although the duration is highly variable.

Diagnosis is standardized by NINCDS criteria which outline subcategories on the basis of certainty of diagnosis. The three categories are possible AD, probable AD and definite AD. A diagnosis of possible AD is assigned when dementia is established through administration of appropriate neuropsychiatric scales (MMSE, Blessed Dementia Scale, etc.) with appropriate age of onset (40–90 years, usually after 65 years), no disturbance of consciousness, deficits in at least two areas of cognition and a progressive deterioration of memory. Possible dementia can also be assigned in the presence of signs that a second dementing process is present (small strokes, etc.) but the second disorder is not sufficiently severe to be the sole cause of the observed cognitive deficits. The main components of a probable AD diagnosis are a progressive dementing illness in the absence of alternative dementing illness. Observations consistent with this diagnosis include progressive deterioration in language, motor skills, or perception; a family history of AD (particularly if it has been confirmed post-mortem); impairment of ability to perform activities of daily living (ADL); normal lumbar puncture and electroencephalogram (EEG) results; serial computerized tomography (CT) scans showing progressive cerebral atrophy. A diagnosis of definite AD is made when there is post-mortem pathological confirmation of AD (as described below), and the patient was assigned a diagnosis of AD in life.

Neuropathology of Alzheimer's disease

The pathological findings of Alzheimer's disease may be readily seen by pathologists upon the use of special histochemical and immunohistochemical stains. However, what has become most apparent is the general lack of correlation between the easily found changes and the clinical stages of dementia. In AD it is possible to identify four major findings on pathological specimens. They include: gross atrophy of the brain, senile plaques, neurofibrillary tangles and amyloid angiopathy.

At autopsy it is often easy to recognize the general atrophy of the frontal and temporal lobes and the moderate enlargement of the lateral ventricles. In addition, the hippocampus can be identified and is often noticeably shrunken.

Tangles, PHFs and tau

Neurofibrillary tangles are identified in the neurons of the neocortex and less commonly in the brainstem neurons of Alzheimer's patients. The tangles are readily identified with silver stains, are fluorescent after treatment with thioflavin S, are birefringent after staining with Congo red and are highlighted by immunohistochemical stains directed to tangle contents. They contain paired helical filaments (PHF) visualized by electron microscopy. These PHFs are different from normal structures such as microtubules and neurofilaments that are identified in uninvolved neurons. The PHFs can be identified within a neuron in intact neurofilbrillary tangles that have outlived their host neuronal cell (ghost tangles), in degenerated neuronal processes near senile plaques and in small thin bundles called 'neuropil threads' in the cortex.

The second major constituent of tangles is an abnormally phosphory-lated microtubule-associated protein, tau (τ). Tau is believed to be a con-stituent or a closely associated protein bound to the PHF. Ubiquitin, a heat shock protein, is also identified within the neurofibrillary tangles of AD. Both ubiquitin and tau can be studied with immunohistochemical methods.

The density of neurofibrillary tangles is often site specific with the Sommer sector of the hippocampus, subiculum (adjacent to the hip-pocampus) and the nucleus basalis of Meynert showing greatest affinity for tangles. Other sites which are often frequently used for study include the frontal and parietal lobes and the superior gyrus of the temporal lobe. The density of neurofibrillary tangles and their anatomical distribution in the transitional zone between the entorhinal allocortex and the temporal isocortex have been correlated with the clinical staging of dementia by Braak and are tightly correlated with cognitive decline in life [3,4] (to a much greater extent than plaques).

Senile plaques and amyloid cores

Senile plaques are often found throughout the neocortex of Alzheimer's patients. They are difficult to identify on routine hematoxylin and eosin stained histological sections of brain tissue. Silver stains and immunohis-tochemical stains for the plaque contents can facilitate their visualization. Plaques are composed of neuronal processes containing neuropil threads and neurofibrillary tangles (as discussed above), astrocytes, microglia cells (brain macrophages) and proteins, mainly the β amyloid peptide. In non-demented aging individuals amyloid can be found in plaques throughout the neocortex. These plaques generally differ from the plaque in AD pathology in that they lack a dense core of amyloid protein. The non-core-containing plaques are often labeled immature or diffuse while those containing cores and associated with tangles and threads are called 'classic'. What is thought to be a late phase of the classic plaque is com-posed of amyloid alone and is called 'burned-out'.

In 1985 Khatchaturian presented a schema that involved both plaque quantity (most often identified by silver stains) and the patient's age to secure a pathological diagnosis of AD; it has since been widely used by neuropathologists. CERAD has published their neuropathological meth-ods for diagnosing AD. Although the assessment process is quite lengthy there has been good correlation between groups of pathologists.

Regardless of the criteria chosen for making the diagnosis of AD, it is critical that historical information on the patient is used along with the pertinent pathological findings. In using the clinical history the pathologist is less likely to overlook one of the rarer causes of dementia in the presence of normal aging changes.

ETIOLOGIC THEORIES OF ALZHEIMER'S DISEASE

To date, no single theory has satisfactorily determined the etiology of the majority of cases of the disease. The evidence provided by epidemiological investigations suggests the most consistent risk factors for AD to be increasing age and a family history of dementia [4]. A meta-analysis, including 11 large case-control studies (ranging from 1980 to 1990) from six different countries, found the main risks significantly associated with AD to be age, positive family history of AD, history of head injury, a history of depression including both recent and distant past episodes, and the presence of Down's syndrome in the family [4]. In addition, this pooled analysis showed smoking to be a dose-dependent protective factor although this is widely debated [5]. Other evidence suggests education, anti-inflammatory use and estrogen replacement therapy as protective factors for AD [6,7]. Recently, data indicating that reserve capacity may be important in risk for AD have been reported, including evidence that AD progression may be related to head size, and early-life linguistic ability may predict AD in late life [8]. More recently genetic epidemiologic studies have begun to correlate environmental influences and genetic risk factors with neuropathological outcomes. Such studies will undoubtedly shed light on the complex etiology of the disorder.

Genetics of Alzheimer's disease

The major etiologic factors responsible for early onset forms of familial AD have been described. Specifically, mutations in three genes, βAPP on chromosome 21 [9–12], PS-1 on chromosome 14 [13], and PS-2 on chromosome 1 [14], have been found to cause the disease in rare AD families. Mutations at codons 717, and 670/671 in the βAPP gene result in the onset of AD near age 55 years, while mutations at over 30 locations in the PS-1 gene result in AD near age 45 years, and a few different mutations in the PS-1 gene result in familial AD with a very wide-ranging age of onset between 50 and 70 years. The mechanisms by which these mutations result in characteristic AD pathology are not completely understood. However, because the clinical and neuropathological features of such cases are not distinguishable from that of late onset disease [15] it is assumed that there is a final common pathway in late and early onset disease and that the mechanism of pathogenesis of early onset AD is relevant to that of late onset AD.

The genetic or environmental risk factors for late onset AD are more heterogeneous than those of early onset AD. No single gene has been identified to have an autosomal dominant relationship to late onset AD in multiply affected families. To date, the only gene convincingly associated with late onset AD, the apolipoprotein E (APOE) gene, is associated with both sporadic and familial cases but does not confer absolute risk for AD [16]. This gene, located on chromosome 19, codes for a lipid carrier protein that associates biologically with both Aβ, cholesterol and estrogen. The three common alleles known to occur in this gene, ε2, ε3, ε4, code for three corresponding protein isoforms, E2, E3, E4. In addition to its association with AD, the ε4 allele of the gene has been found to confer risk for atherosclerosis and coronary artery disease (CAD) [17,18], and has also been suggested to influence mortality through its role as a cholesterol transporter. It has also been reported to have a significantly increased frequency among ischemic heart and stroke cases [19] although it is generally assumed that the mechanism underlying these disorders is different from the mechanism underlying the risk for AD.

The ε4 allele of the APOE gene confers risk for the development (or earlier clinical manifestation) of AD in a dose-dependent way (homozygotes have the highest risk, while heterozygotes are also at increased risk over non-carriers) [16,20]. However, this APOE variant does not confer absolute risk for AD, as evidenced by the proportion of ε4 carriers who do not develop the disease, even by age 85 years, and by the proportion of non-ε4 carriers who do develop AD. Also, among familial cases of late onset AD, the risk conferred by ε4 cannot account for all of the risk due to family history of the disease [21], suggesting other familial factors (genetic or environmental) must contribute to the etiology of the disease. This invites the investigation of other genes that may be associated with the disease in a similar way to APOE. One further area of intense investigation is whether different APOE alleles confer differential response to pharmacotherapy. Many large scale clinical trials of anti-AD drugs include an APOE genotyping component.

βAPP metabolism and Alzheimer's disease neuropathology

The discovery of genetic mutations triggering early onset AD has driven the theories of AD pathogenesis. The discovery of genetic linkage between βAPP mutants and AD, in addition to the preponderance of Aβ (a metabolite of βAPP) in AD plaques, and the occurrence of AD pathology in Down's syndrome (where overexpression of the βAPP gene is assumed) has highlighted βAPP as a central molecule in the disease process. βAPP is a 770 amino acid transmembrane glycoprotein which, while expressed nearly ubiquitously, achieves its highest expression in neuronal and glial cells. Within βAPP, β-amyloid is located in the transmembrane domain and is normally [22] cleaved variably to produce a protein between 39 and 43 amino acids in length ($A\beta_{1-39} - A\beta_{1-43}$).

Processing of βAPP occurs through three common, normally occurring pathways, and involves at least three secretase cleavage sites (α, β, and γ). The first pathway involves cleavage of the transmembrane βAPP protein at the α-secretase site within the Aβ domain, resulting in a large (> 100 kDa) N-terminal fragment, APPs (which is secreted by the cell) and also identified as protease nexin II. Cleavage at this site precludes Aβ peptide formation, as shown in Fig. 5.1. The second pathway utilizes the endosomal-lysosomal cellular pathways to clear a 10–22 kDa C-terminal fragment which includes the entire Aβ domain, and could possibly result in release of Aβ [23]. The final pathway involves cleavage of APP at two sites, the β and γ secretase sites as shown in Fig 5.1, which results in secretion of the Aβ fragment. The β-secretase cleavage results in C-terminal heterogeneity of the Aβ fragments which is either due to the existence of more than one γ-secretase or to the non-specificity of the cleavage. Recently Klafki *et al.* [24] have suggested that there are two γ-secretases. The exact identity of the secretases has yet to be determined. Neither is it known whether there are specific secretases for βAPP or whether these enzymes cleave several molecules. In advance of the identification of these secretases certain substances have already been identified that either increase the α cleavage or decrease the β or γ cleavages and reduce βAPP processing into Aβ.

The locations of the three secretase sites on the APP protein approximately co-localize with the location of genetic mutations resulting in AD. The double mutation (670/671) [12] is located in the region coding for the

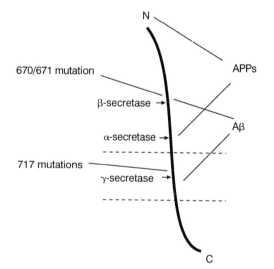

Fig. 5.1 βAPP transmembrane protein with processing cleavage sites and Alzheimer's mutations.

area immediately before the N terminus of the Aβ domain (near the β-secretase site) and results in five to eight times increased Aβ production [25]. The other missense mutations in βAPP are localized just beyond the C terminus of Aβ (near the γ-secretase site), and result in production of normal amounts of Aβ, but in a longer form (Aβ$_{1-42}$ rather than Aβ$_{1-40}$) [26]. This longer form of Aβ forms aggregates more rapidly, and may therefore be more amyloidogenic. A third site of mutation in this gene (resulting in Dutch amyloid angiopathy) is located within the Aβ domain and results in the production of an Aβ peptide with an alternative amino acid sequence [27]. Finally, the PS-1 and PS-2 mutations also result in a shift of βAPP processing towards an increase in Aβ$_{1-42}$ in brains of transgenic mice [28] and in increased serum levels of Aβ$_{1-42}$ in AD patients carrying such mutations [29].

Because all the early onset genetic errors result in a shift of processing towards either more Aβ production or the production of longer Aβ fragments (or both) therapies which correct this shift are being designed. Some new pharmacotherapies are being aimed simply at decreasing the total amount of Aβ produced by altering secretase activity. Other therapies may be aimed at specifically inhibiting the γ-secretase cut that results in the Aβ$_{1-42}$ peptide. In this regard it is of some interest that recently evidence has emerged that there are distinct γ-secretases resulting in the Aβ$_{1-40}$ and Aβ$_{1-42}$ fragments [24]. Other therapeutic opportunities may arise from the physicochemical characteristics of Aβ which promote its aggregation and deposition. It is hypothesized that the common pathological consequence of excess Aβ$_{1-42}$ production is Aβ aggregation and deposition [29] although it remains a possibility that this is a secondary phenomenon loosely associated with neurotoxicity. It is the case, though, that the toxicity of Aβ fragments in cell culture is associated with its aggregation state (below) but the clinical relevance of this finding *in vitro* has yet to be established. For instance, serum or CSF Aβ$_{1-42}$ levels are not raised in the common late onset AD.

Aβ toxicity

Aβ toxicity in neuronal cell cultures has been shown to be time, dose, and fragment length dependent [30]. Each of these factors favors aggregation and it is now generally thought that dimeric and higher order organization into fibrils is a requisite for rapid cell death in culture conditions [31]. In the same conditions but with lower (and more physiologic) doses, Aβ peptides may be trophic. It should be borne in mind that all the aggregation/toxicity data are derived from extremely high peptide doses (1–100 μM) applied over a period of hours and days. The extent to which this mimics a 10–15 year process where normal physiologic levels (at least in serum) are at least three orders of magnitude less must be questioned.

Aβ aggregation is thought to be toxic to neurons via oxy-radical production which results in disruption of ATP-ase dependent pumps [32] with consequent loss of calcium homeostasis. Furthermore, the presence of Aβ in cell culture can enhance glutamate-induced excitotoxic death [33]. Consistent with this idea is the observation that prevention of calcium influx can prevent neuronal toxicity in cell culture. The nature of Aβ-induced cell death is currently controversial, although increasing evidence suggests apoptotic cell death [34].

Normal roles for βAPP and Aβ

Compared with Aβ pathogenicity the normal roles of βAPP and Aβ are far less understood. Some evidence suggests APPs may play a role in cell adhesion [35], in neurite outgrowth [36], or in synaptogenesis [37]. Recent evidence indicates that the secreted APPs is a trophic factor with neuronal survival and protective activity *in vitro* and *in vivo* against a variety of insults [38]. The domain of APPs responsible for those activities has been mapped to the central region of the molecule, from Ala319 to Met335. A peptide representing the trophic domain of APP increased memory retention in rats [39] and protected them from neurological damage after ischemic insult [40]. In addition, APP expressed in transgenic mice protected neurons from gp120-induced toxicity [41]. The data available indicated that the trophic effect of APPs is mediated by a receptor whose activity is involved in the regulation of calcium homeostasis [38]. APPs has also been implicated in aspects of the immune system and may confer protection to the CNS via these mechanisms [42]. The increased Aβ formation in AD may represent impaired formation of APPs and loss of one of these normal functions, given the reciprocal relation between APPs formation and Aβ formation.

Abnormal phosphorylation of tau and NFT formation

Tau is a microtubule-associated protein which is localized to the axonal compartment and is involved in axonal transport and microtubule elongation and nucleation. Repeat sequences within tau bind to microtubules (Fig. 5.2), and protect tubulin from disassembly. Tau's affinity for tubulin and ability to regulate outgrowth are at least partly controlled by phosphorylation, which is altered in AD neurons. Excessive phosphorylation of tau at Ser/Thr-sites in AD brains results in the aggregation of tau bound to itself in anti-parallel dimers which form paired helical filaments (PHF), which then precludes tau–microtubule binding. These are wound around each other with cross-over repeats, but do not show obvious alpha-helix or beta-sheet secondary structure.

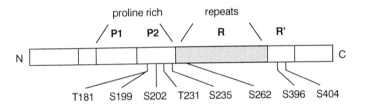

Fig. 5.2 Tau protein with abnormally phosphorylated Ser and Thr sites shown. The repeat region which binds to tubulin is shaded.

Although the four repeat sequences within tau are the actual binding sites to tubulin, the presence of the P1 and R' flanking regions appears to be more important in tubulin-binding affinity than specific repeats or number of repeats [for a review see ref. 43]. It is within these flanking regions that most of the abnormal phosphorylation sites associated with AD exist (see Fig. 5.2), although induced phosphorylation at these sites does not severely inhibit tau–tubulin binding. However, the Ser262 site within the first repeat sequence of tau is uniquely phosphorylated in AD cases and not in controls, and phosphorylation of this site *in vitro* virtually stops tau–microtubule binding [43]. There is some inconsistency in these data, given that the tau repeat flanking regions appear important in tight binding to microtubules yet their phosphorylation seems to have trivial effects on binding, but phosphorylation within the first repeat can very strongly influence binding. This area has yet to be clarified and knowledge of the tertiary structure of tau or tubulin may be helpful in this regard.

The state of phosphorylation of tau depends on the relative activities of protein kinases and phosphatases. Most of the abnormally phosphorylated sites can be phosphorylated by several kinases (MAP kinase, GSK3, cdk5 and others) and dephosphorylated by protein phosphatases 2A and 2B [44]. It appears that the balance between phosphorylation and dephosphorylation may be disrupted in PHF tau, leading to the hyperphosphorylation at these sites [45]. This is supported by the observation of decreased amounts of phosphatases in AD cases [46] and increased tau phosphorylation by phosphatase inhibitors *in vitro* [47].

APOE involvement in Alzheimer's disease neuropathology

The discovery of genetic association between AD and the APOE gene has led to investigation into ways that APOE could play a background role in AD pathogenesis. The observation that APOE co-localizes with Aβ in plaques gave rise to a possibility that APOE binds to amyloid directing plaque formation – a hypothesis which is supported by binding studies indicating E4 binds preferentially to Aβ over either the E3 or E2 isoforms [48]. APOE has also been shown to form monofibrillar structures with β-amyloid, again with the E4 isoform having a greater tendency to do this than the E3 isoform [49]. Through its role as a lipid transport molecule, and as the primary lipoprotein expressed in the brain, APOE has also been implicated in neural regeneration by redistributing lipids to neurons during extension and to specialized cells during remyelination. *In vitro* studies have shown that cholesterol-associated APOE stimulates neural branching, and that this occurs in an isoform-specific manner – E3 shows greater stimulation of growth relative to E4 [50]. These observations might suggest a role for APOE isoform specific promotion of insolubility and deposition of Aβ in AD pathogenesis – although this idea is disputed. Other theories for the role of APOE E4 concern its ability to promote PHF formation [51]. In contrast to E4, it has been suggested that E3 slows the rate of tau phosphorylation and thereby slows the self assembly into PHFs. APOE E4 does not bind tau and therefore cannot prevent slow PHF formation. It was also noted that hyperphosphorylated tau cannot bind APOE, suggesting that once PHF formation has begun any protective role by APOE may be lost.

The finding that APOE can resist Aβ-induced oxidative stress in an isoform-specific manner (E2 > E3 > E4) [52] suggests an alternative mechanism by which APOE isoforms might influence the AD process. This suggestion is particularly attractive as it seems to offer a link between Aβ and APOE in terms of production of and resistance to oxidative stresses (and therefore the aging process). At this time it is not known which of the various mechanisms suggested for APOE influence on AD are important and which are not.

Cholinergic system in Alzheimer's disease

Although a number of neurotransmitter systems are altered in AD brains, the cholinergic system appears to be the most severely affected as exemplified by massive loss of cholinergic neurons in the hippocampus and cholinergic enzymes in the cerebral cortex. In addition, since the 1980s, learning and memory have been intimately associated with the cholinergic system. Coyle and colleagues adapted the Bartus acetylcholine (ACh) theory of memory to AD specifically for three reasons: (1) there is a notable loss of acetylcholine (and the enzyme that produces it) in AD patients, (2) there is a correlation between biochemical measures of ACh systems and clinical decline in AD patients, and (3) there is loss of basal forebrain neurons in AD patients [53].

More recently, molecular associations between βAPP and the cholinergic system have been identified, specifically that muscarinic receptors may mediate APPs secretion. Nitsch *et al.* [54], for instance, showed that activation of the m1 muscarinic receptor can stimulate the secretion of APPs through the α-secretase pathway with a concomitant reduction of Aβ release. Thus, loss of ACh and downregulation of muscarinic receptor activation could result in increased Aβ release. Also, muscarinic receptor activation and signal transduction via G proteins has been shown to be disrupted by $A\beta_{1-40}$ and $A\beta_{25-35}$ [55]. Exposure of rodent fetal cortical neurons to these peptides caused an attenuation of carbachol-induced GTPase activity without affecting muscarinic receptor ligand binding parameters. These effects of Aβ peptides on carbachol-induced GTPase activity and calcium release were attenuated by antioxidants, suggesting the generation of free radicals as an intermediate step.

From these and other related findings four potential pharmacological treatments have been proposed: use of ACh precursors, use of ACh releasers, direct-acting ACh agonists, and cholinesterase inhibitors. In the first group, choline precursor drugs were suggested, specifically lecithin, as a way of increasing the amount of extracellular choline, a precursor to ACh. In clinical trials, this approach was relatively unsuccessful [56]. A second, and much more promising approach used inhibitors of the enzyme acetylcholinesterase (ChEIs), which hydrolyzes acetylcholine, increasing the overall amount of ACh at the synaptic cleft. Early studies included the use of physostigmine, which showed promise but has a short half-life, making it impractical for the long-term treatment of AD. Many other ChEIs have been tested, but to date, only tacrine (brand name Cognex) and donetevil HCI (brand name Aricept) have been approved by the FDA. The use of nicotinic ACh receptor (nAChR) agonists is a growing area of clinical activity in AD pharmacotherapy and is discussed below. It is known that activation of the α-7 nAChR subtype can induce anti-apoptotic cytoprotection in both neuronal and non-neuronal systems [57]. Nicotinic agonists can also prevent neuronal cell death induced by glutamate and Aβ [58].

Inflammation in Alzheimer's disease

Inflammatory markers have been observed frequently and ubiquitously in AD patients leading to an etiologic theory of immune-mediated autodestructive processes. In particular, it has been suggested that inflammatory reactions are required to convert the presence of an amyloid burden into a pathologic process. McGeer and Rogers [59] have shown a poor inflammatory response in individuals with high AD pathology but no cognitive features. However, in AD individuals, elements of the immune system are significantly increased over normal controls and over non-demented controls with high amounts of plaques or tangles. For instance, a large number of immune system proteins occur in association with characteristic AD lesions, including enhanced levels of immunoglobulin receptors, complement receptors, and major histocompatibility complex (MHC) glycoproteins on reactive microglia: increased cytokine production; T lymphocyte infiltration tissue; complement protein fixation to plaques, tangles, and dystrophic neurites; and appearance of complement inhibitors appearing on damaged neurons and their processes. Also, antibodies to complement proteins of the classic pathway densely label pathologic elements in AD tissue, but not in control brains. Two other proteins found in amyloid plaques are also associated with immunoreaction: alpha-1-antichymotrypsin, and alpha-2-macroglobulin. These are both associated with the inflammatory acute phase response.

Oxidative stress and damage in Alzheimer's disease

Harman has extended his free radical theory of aging to the pathogenesis of AD, stating that an imbalance of naturally occurring free radicals may provide the background for subsequent neurodegeneration and cellular death, possibly by disrupting calcium homeostasis within the cell. Sustained increases in cellular Ca^{2+} disrupt the cytoskeleton and activate calcium-dependent catabolic enzymes. This theory has lacked specific detail as applied to AD, although in recent years direct links between βAPP or Aβ and free radical damage and other constituents of AD pathology have been made. Mattson [38] linked altered processing of βAPP to disruption of neuronal calcium homeostasis, leading to an excitotoxic mechanism of cell death in AD. As noted above, a major pathway of βAPP metabolism results in the release of secreted forms of βAPP. APPs can protect neurons against excitotoxic or ischemic insults by stabilizing the intracellular calcium concentration [60]. Obversely, Aβ peptides can disrupt calcium homeostasis and render neurons vulnerable to metabolic or excitotoxic injury. Differences in expression of antioxidant enzymes (detected by immunocytochemical techniques) between AD and normals support the idea of increased oxidative stress as a mechanism in the pathogenesis of AD [61].

SITES FOR PHARMACOLOGIC INTERVENTION

Regulation of APP processing

If the observations above are verified, and $A\beta_{1-42}$ is the key pathogenic species in AD, a key question is how does it cause the disease process? $A\beta_{1-42}$ is less soluble and might be pathogenic by virtue of its propensity to aggregate, form Aβ fibrils and precipitate in the brain parenchyma. Neuronal loss, in this model, is due to toxicity of $A\beta_{1-42}$ or due to the negative consequences of anti-inflammatory cascades triggered by its deposition.

The neurotrophic and neuroprotective activity of APPs opens new therapeutic avenues in AD. The trophic activity is retained in a small peptide in the central region of the protein, and is mediated by a receptor system. Pharmacological agents designed either to activate this receptor or to stimulate secretion of APPs through the α-secretase pathway may represent viable drug candidates for treatment and/or prevention.

Stimulation of a number of systems via cell surface receptors results in increase production of APPs and therefore a relative reduction of Aβ fragments. Known receptors that, when stimulated, increase APPs secretion are the m1 and m3 acetylcholine receptors, $5HT_{2a}$ and $5HT_{2c}$ and the glutamatergic mGlu R1 receptors. All these receptors are G-protein coupled, and some tyrosine kinase-coupled receptor systems also increase the secretion of APPs. For instance, nerve growth factor upregulates APP [62] and stimulates APPs secretion [63] as do cytokines [62]. These and other first messenger systems and their receptors offer potential therapeutic sites with quite conventional pharmacology.

For several reasons it can be argued that the production of deposited amyloid is not central to the disease process although clearly the genetic evidence implicates the βAPP gene and its product. An alternative theory is that the mutations in the gene alter the normal function of the gene and its metabolites. In this scenario, normalization of βAPP processing would therefore remain a desirable therapeutic aim whether amyloidogenic metabolism or change of function of APP is central to the disease process.

Regulation of tau phosphorylation

Two therapeutic strategies related to the pathologic evidence of NFT formation in AD brains are the activation of phosphatases and the inactivation of kinases responsible for the regulation of tau phosphorylation. Given the unique phosphorylation of Ser262 among AD patients, and its location within a repeat sequence and apparent association with tubulin binding, it is important to investigate the possible kinases responsible for phosphorylation of this site specifically, or phosphatases helpful in specific dephosphorylation at this site.

To date, many proline-directed kinases (MAP kinase, GSK-3, cdk2, cdk5, etc.) have been shown to phosphorylate tau at several sites within the flanking regions (both in normal and AD forms of tau) [64]. All of these sites can be dephosphorylated by phosphatases PP-2A or PP-2B (calcineurin) [65]. In addition, other non-Ser-Pro motifs can be phosphorylated by CaM kinase, PKA, PKC or casein kinase II [66], and these can all be dephosphorylated by PP-2A or PP-2B. None of these, however, was responsible for phosphorylation at a site that significantly altered tau–tubulin binding. Furthermore, manipulation of kinases with a wide range of substrates could result in the disruption of many other cellular activities. Recently, however, specific phosphorylation of the Ser262 site has been demonstrated by a novel kinase – MARK (MAP/microtubule affinity-regulating kinase) [67]. Manipulation of this enzyme may represent a therapeutic opportunity, yet further work in this area is required.

An additional target for therapeutic intervention may be increased activation of the protein phosphatases 2A and 2B. Manipulation of these is thought not as likely to induce other cellular problems [68], and the specific dephosphorylation of Ser262 would be ideal.

Cholinergic therapies

Drugs acting on the cholinergic system are differentiated by their chemical classes and their mechanism of inhibition of cholinesterase: carbamates represented by physostigmine (reviewed above) and SDZ ENA 713; tetrahydroaminoacridine represented by tacrine; and benzylpiperidines represented by E20 20.

Given the several lines of evidence showing reduced acetylcholine receptor stimulation in AD and the specific links suggesting nAChR stimulation might enhance cognitive abilities (above) nAChR agonists represent a potential therapeutic family of compounds. GTS-21 (2, 4 dimethoxybenzylidene anabaseine) is representative of novel nAChR agonists with receptor subtype specificity [69]. Two primary metabolites of GTS-21 are α7-nAChR agonists. GTS-21 is known to enhance cognitive tasks in several animal species and is under clinical trial in AD.

Management of inflammatory pathways

Whether an inflammatory response is solely due to a reaction to Aβ deposition or other elements of pathology is not known. The data do at least point to relatively immediate pragmatic strategies for treatment, as many anti-inflammatory drugs with well-established low levels of adverse reactions are already available. Clinical trials comparing treatment with non-steroidal anti-inflammatory drugs (NSAIDs) and measures of cognitive decline are currently underway with as yet inconclusive but apparently promising results [70]. Current prospective trials are underway at several clinics, but results may be timely as there are many problems with conducting clinical trials of such a ubiquitously used medication.

Management of oxidative stress and damage

Much of the rationale for therapeutic intervention in free radical imbalances that occur in AD remains theoretical. In Down's syndrome, for instance, the pathology of AD is found as individuals age into the third and fourth decade. Busciglio and Yanker [71] reported that cortical neurons from fetal Down's syndrome degenerate and undergo apoptosis as they age compared with age-matched normal neurons which remain viable. Free-radical scavengers or catalase prevent degeneration of Down's syndrome neurons. There is also direct evidence that $A\beta_{1-40}$ generates free radicals during incubation in cell-free aqueous solution [72]. The translation of these findings to clinically relevant and disease-specific therapies has not yet occurred.

The direct use of the superoxide dismutases, catalases and glutathione peroxidase, the naturally occurring antioxidants, presents difficulties mostly in terms of drug delivery. Clinically viable alternatives include the antioxidant vitamins and spin trap compounds like *N-tert*-butyl-α-phenylnitrone (PBN). Such compounds are now going into clinical trials in a range of neurodegenerative disorders.

Additional potential therapies

Estrogen

It has been noted that Alzheimer's disease has a lower prevalence in women treated post-menopausally with estrogen replacement therapy. This led to speculation that estrogen therapy might be protective against AD. At the molecular level there is some support for this; 17 β-estradiol increases the amount of APPs cleavage from the βAPP molecule and Aβ-induced oxidative stress can be opposed by 17 β-estradiol. Clinical trials of estrogen are required to provide direct evidence for a role of estrogens in: (1) the prevention of Alzheimer's disease, (2) slowing of the rate of progression of the disease, or (3) other interactions, for instance with APOE genotype. Such trials are currently underway at many sites.

Excitotoxic amino acid receptor block

$A\beta_{25-35}$ has been shown to induce excitatory bursts in current-clamped individual neurons. This electrical activity can be blocked by NMDA glutamate receptor antagonists [73]. Electron paramagnetic resonance studies show that intact mitochondria generate hydroxyl radicals when exposed to increased calcium and sodium levels [74]. Busciglio *et al.* [71] showed that in 36 day old human fetal cultures Aβ toxicity was not inhibited by excitatory amino acid receptor antagonists. They concluded that Aβ toxicity did not directly involve excitotoxic amino acid receptors. It has also been shown that Aβ peptides destabilize calcium homeostasis and thereby render human cortical neurons vulnerable to excitotoxic insult [33]. Note that early studies of NMDA receptor agonists as potential treatments for AD via stimulation of long-term potentiation were disappointing, consistent with the notion that stimulation would be harmful in this condition. Clinical studies have begun to investigate the usefulness of NMDA receptor antagonists primarily in stroke and head injury studies and it remains to be seen whether clinical trials extend to Alzheimer's disease where the role of these systems in disease pathogenesis is more obscure.

Calcium channel blockers

As raised intracellular calcium levels may be a final common event in several pathways of neurodegeneration the potential therapeutic use of calcium channel blockers in AD continues to be seriously considered. As mentioned above, $A\beta$ and APPs seem to have opposing roles in the maintenance of calcium homeostasis in cortical neurons. Calcium is central to excitotoxic cell death and is linked to the activation of nitric oxide synthase and the production of other free radicals via a variety of systems [74]. Raised intracellular calcium is also a consequence of free radical activity. Nimodipine, a dihydropyridine with calcium channel-blocking properties, can block depolarization-induced intracellular calcium increases in rat hippocampal neurons. In addition, intracellular calcium levels raised by $A\beta_{25-25}$ exposure can also be blocked by nimodipine. In an early randomized double blind trial of 227 AD cases treated with low-dose nimodipine [75], the author concluded that there was deterioration across several cognitive and social parameters.

VASCULAR DEMENTIA

The main alternative cause of dementia is vascular pathology resulting in infarction and ischemia. The histopathologic features of ischemia are determined by the severity and time since the ischemic event. The earliest changes noted include eosinophilic neurons and an infiltration by polymorphonuclear neutrophils which is then followed by macrophage infiltration. Late changes include reactive astrocytosis and cavitation. Less critical ischemic events may involve only a loss of neurons and mild astrocytosis in the gray matter or thinning of the white matter (with visible loss of myelin), referred to as rarefaction. These changes are uniform regardless of the cause of the infarction.

Cortical dementias include multi-infarct dementia, single-infarct dementia and distal-field dementia. 'Multi-infarct dementia' is used to suggest a dementia which has been cumulative in nature, due to the superimposition of many ischemic strokes, spread out both in time and space. Multi-infarct dementia has most often been attributed to cerebral embolic events (originating in the heart, basilar or carotid arteries) or thrombosis of large or medium-sized intracranial arteries. Atherosclerosis and cardiac arrhythmias are the usual predisposing diseases. The risk factors for multi-infarct dementia include hypertension, hypercholesterolemia, diabetes mellitus, obesity and smoking.

'Single-infarct dementia' or 'strategic-infarct dementia' occurs when a single cerebrovascular event is determined to be the cause of dementia. The term 'strategic' relates to the precise determination of the intellectual impairment by a single stroke; the limbic system, association cortex and deep gray nuclei, along with their white matter pathways, are frequently involved. Single-infarct and multi-infarct dementia have similar risk factors.

The brain has multiple areas which are especially vulnerable to hypoperfusion when there is a decrease in systemic blood pressure. Ischemia with classic histopathology and neuroimaging can be identified in these areas that are often referred to as 'watershed regions'. These regions lie between the major terminal branches of the main cerebral and cerebellar arteries. The end arterioles of these major branches are unable to autoregulate and compensate for collateral blood flow in the hypotensive state. The frontal lobe, fronto-parietal region, occipital lobe and cerebellum may all be involved bilaterally and simultaneous distal-field dementia is one term used to describe a dementia with hypotensive pathophysiology and may be used regardless of the number of ischemic lesions.

Subcortical dementia may also be classified as multi-infarct or single-infarct and include, in addition, Binswanger's disease. Multi-infarct dementia, when subcortical, suggests that the ischemic lesions are confined to the basal ganglia. The pathological gross and microscopic picture is often of multiple small cavitated lesions with a thin gliotic lining. Each individual infarct is called a lacune, and the combination of many is termed 'etat lacunare'. Hypertension with subsequent atherosclerosis of the basilar artery and/or arteriosclerosis of the penetrating vessels of the deep gray and white matter is most often implicated in this disease. Single-infarct dementia, or strategic-infarct dementia of the subcortical brain, most often involves the thalamus, caudate or internal capsule.

Binswanger's disease is somewhat synonymous with the neuroimaging term 'leukoaraiosis' and is associated with reduced cerebral blood flow to the periventricular white matter as its cause. The histopathologic changes of small vessels include circumferential thickening of the vessel wall, hyaline deposition and intimal proliferation. As described earlier, the affected white matter shows thinning of the myelin sheaths and mild astrogliosis. Etiologic theories include both arteriosclerosis and hypotension combining to cause the periventricular end arterioles to receive suboptimal flow. The debate in recent years is often over whether pure 'subcortical' dementia can be caused by this periventricular white matter disease, as the neuroimaging findings of leukoaraiosis are quite common in elderly patients both with and without dementia, and are often seen in combination with other clinically diagnosed dementias. One group of experimental medications which may be useful in conditions where dementia occurs due to obvious vascular pathology are the calcium channel blockers. As well as having direct cerebrovascular dilating activity [for a review see ref. 76] some of these medications protect neurons from excitotoxic cell death by opposing raised intracellular free calcium levels at least in animal models [77]. Administered prior to ischemia in experimental middle cerebral artery occlusion paradigms, nimodipine can significantly reduce infarct sizes and can reduce post-ischemic cerebral hypoperfusion. Such drugs have also been shown to enhance learning in aging animals [78]. Because of the broad roles of these medications they are being tried in a wide range of dementias due to several causes including vascular dementia, AD and dementia due to mixed etiology. A preliminary trial of patients with cognitive impairment and leukoaraiosis may show promising results.

Cerebral amyloid angiopathy – as related to aging and dementia

Amyloid angiopathy has been described in both the elderly and in genetically susceptible families. The genetic forms of cerebral amyloid angiopathy are caused by several amyloidogenic proteins, including amyloid β, transthyretin (TTR, prealbumin), cystatin C and protease-resistant prion protein.

Some amyloid deposition (stars) occurs in and around the smooth muscle layers of vessels. In capillaries and precapillaries Aβ fibrils accumulate in the basal lamina. The amyloid deposition in the wall of the vessel causes degeneration of endothelial cells and in many vessels obliteration of their lumen. In areas of amyloid angiopathy, extensive degeneration of the neurons without neurofibrillary changes is observed. This pathology is probably caused mainly by local ischemia, raising the question of hypoperfusion as a component of the AD process. Three types of cells produce amyloid fibrils in the vascular wall: perivascular cells enclosed within the basal lamina, migrating perivascular cells and perivascular microglial cells. Amyloid forms thick semicircular, circular or tuberous deposits in the vascular wall. There is evidence that Aβ fibril formation takes place in the vascular basement membrane. It is likely that some of the pharmacotherapies designed to reduce Aβ formation in brain parenchyma will also be helpful in reducing Aβ burden and damage in amyloid angiopathy.

CONCLUSION

While existing therapy focuses on the known neurotransmitter defects, steady advances in the understanding of specific pathogenic mechanisms of Alzheimer's disease are resulting in new therapies directed towards abnormal β-APP and tau processing. It is likely that as our molecular understanding of the disease process becomes more clear, correspondingly specific molecular therapies will emerge. In addition, many more insights need to be gained as to the nature of the vascular dementias and their relationship to Alzheimer's disease. With such correlation in mind, it can be expected that in the next 5–10 years, existing medications (with primary indications other than dementia) are likely to be tried alone and in combination in these disorders.

REFERENCES

1. Hsaio, K., Chapman, P., Nilsen, S., *et al.* (1996) Correlative memory deficits, Aβ elevation, and amyloid plaques in transgenic mice. *Science*, **274**, 99–102.
2. Ernst, R. and Hay, J. (1994) The US economic and social costs of Alzheimer's disease revisited. *American Journal of Public Health*, **84**, 1261–1264.
3. Braak, H. and Braak, E. (1994) In *Neurodegenerative diseases*. D. Calne *et al.*, Eds, pp. 585–613. Philadelphia: W.B. Saunders Co.
4. Van Duijn, C.M., Stijnen, T. and Hofman, A. (1991) Risk factors for Alzheimer's disease: overview of the EURODEM collaborative re-analysis of case-control studies. *International Journal of Epidemiology*, **20** (Suppl. 2), S4–S12.
5. Graves, A.B., van Duijn, C.M., Chandra, V., *et al.* (1991) Alcohol and tobacco consumption as risk factors for Alzheimer's disease: a collaborative reanalysis of case-control studies. *International Journal of Epidemiology*, **20** (S2), S48–S57.
6. McGeer, P., Schulzer, M. and McGeer, E. (1996) Arthritis and anti-inflammatory agents as possible protective factors for Alzheimer's disease. *Neurology*, **47**, 425–432.
7. Tang, M.-X., Jacobs, D., Stern, Y., *et al.* (1996) Effect of oestrogen during menopause on risk and age at onset of Alzheimer's disease. *Lancet*, **348**, 429–432.
8. Graves, A.B., Mortimer, J., Larson, A., *et al.* (1996) Head circumference as a measure of cognitive reserve association with severity of impairment in Alzheimer's disease. *British Journal of Psychiatry*, **169**, 86–92.
9. Chartier Harlin, M.C., Crawford, F., Houlden, H.C., *et al.* (1991) Early onset Alzheimer's disease caused by mutations at codon 717 of the β-amyloid precursor protein gene. *Nature*, **353**, 844–846.
10. Goate, A., Chartier-Harlin, M.C., Mullan, M., *et al.* (1991) Segregation of a missense mutation in the amyloid precursor protein gene with familial Alzheimer's disease. *Nature*, **349**, 704–706.
11. Murrell, J., Farlow, M., Ghetti, B., *et al.* (1991) A mutation in the amyloid precursor protein associated with hereditary Alzheimer's disease. *Science*, **254**, 97–99.
12. Mullan, M., Crawford, F., Axelman, K., *et al.* (1992) A pathogenic mutation for probable Alzheimer's disease in the APP gene at the N-terminus of β-amyloid. *Nature Genetics*, **1**, 345–347.
13. Levy-Lahad, E., Waxco, W., Poorkaj, P., *et al.* (1995) Candidate gene for the chromosome 1 familial Alzheimer's disease locus. *Science*, **269**, 973–977.
14. Sherrington, R., Rogaev, E., Liang, Y., *et al.* (1995) Cloning of a gene bearing mis-sense mutations in early onset familial Alzheimer's disease. *Nature*, **375**, 754–760.

15. Mullan, M., Tsuji, S., Miki, T., *et al.* (1993) Clinical comparison of Alzheimer's disease in pedigrees with the codon 717 ValIle mutation in the amyloid precursor protein gene. *Neurobiology of Aging*, **14**, 407–419.

16. Mullan, M., Scibelli, P., Duara, R., *et al.* (1997) Familial and population based studies of APOE and AD. *Annals of the New York Academy of Science*, **802**, 16–26.

17. Miida, T. (1990) Apolipoprotein E phenotype in patients with coronary heart disease. *Experimental Medicine*, **160**, 177–187.

18. Davignon, J., Gregg, R. and Sing, C. (1988) Apolipoprotein E polymorphism and atherosclerosis. *Arteriosclerosis*, **8**, 1–21.

19. Pedro-Botet, J., Senti, M., Nogues, X., *et al.* (1992) Lipoprotein and apolipoprotein profile in men with ischemic stroke. Role of lipoprotein (a), triglyceride-rich lipoproteins and apolipoprotein E polymorphism. *Stroke*, **23**, 1556–1562.

20. Corder, E., Saunders, A., Strittmatter, W., *et al.* (1993) Gene dose of apolipoprotein E type 4 allele and the risk of Alzheimer's disease in late onset families. *Science*, **261**, 921–923.

21. Jarvik, G.P., Larson, E.B., Goddard, K., *et al.* (1996) Influence of apolipoprotein E genotype on the transmission of Alzheimer disease in a community-based sample. *American Journal of Human Genetics*, **58**, 191–200.

22. Haass, C., Schlossmacher, A., Hung, A.Y. *et al.* (1992) Amyloid-B peptide is produced by cultured cells during normal metabolism. *Nature*, **359**, 322–325.

23. Haass, C., Koo, E.H., Mellon, A., *et al.* (1992) Targeting of cell-surface b-amyloid precursor protein to lysosomes: alternative processing into amyloidogenic fragments. *Nature*, **357**, 500–503.

24. Klafki, H.W., Abramowski, D., Swoboda, R., *et al.* (1996) The carboxyl termini of beta-amyloid peptides 1–40 and 1–42 are generated by distinct gamma-secretase activities. *Journal of Biological Chemistry*, **271**, 28655–28659.

25. Citron, M., Oltersdorf, T., Haass, C., *et al.* (1992) Mutation of the b-amyloid precursor protein in familial AD increases b-amyloid production. *Nature*, **360**, 672–674.

26. Suzuki, N., Cheung, T.T., Cai, X.D., *et al.* (1994) An increased percentage of long amyloid beta secreted by familial amyloid b precursor protein (BAPP717) mutants. *Science*, **264**, 1336–1340.

27. Haass, C., Hung, A.Y., Selkoe, D.J., *et al.* (1994) Mutations associated with a locus for familial Alzheimer's disease result in alternative processing of amyloid b precursor protein. *Journal of Biological Chemistry*, **269**, 1–8.

28. Duff, K., Eckman, C., Zehr, C., *et al.* (1996) Increased amyloid-β42(43) in brains of mice expressing mutant presenilin 1. *Nature*, **383**, 710–713.

29. Scheuner, D., Eckman, C., Jensen, M., *et al.* (1996) Secreted amyloid b-protein similar to that in the senile plaques of Alzheimer's disease is increased *in vivo* by the presenilin 1 and 2 and APP mutations linked to familial Alzheimer's disease. *Nature Medicine*, **2**, 864–870.

30. Iversen, L.L., Mortishire-Smith, R.J., Pollack, S.J., *et al.* (1995) The toxicity in vitro of beta-amyloid protein. *Biochemical Journal*, **311**, 1–16.

31. Howlett, D.R., Jennings, K.H., Lee, D.C., *et al.* (1995) Aggregation state and neurotoxic properties of Alzheimer beta-amyloid peptide. *Neurodegeneration*, **4**, 23–32.

32. Mark, R.J., Hensley, K., Butterfield, D.A., *et al.* (1995) Amyloid beta peptide impairs ion-motive ATPase activities: evidence for a role in loss of neuronal Ca^{2+} homeostasis and cell death. *Journal of Neuroscience*, **15**, 6239–6249.

33. Mattson, M., Cheng, B., Davis, D., *et al.* (1992) Beta amyloid peptides destabilize calcium homeostasis and render human cortical neurons vulnerable to excitotoxicity. *Journal of Neuroscience*, **12**, 379–389.

34. Cotman, C.W. and Anderson, A.J. (1995) A potential role for apoptosis in neurodegeneration and Alzheimer's disease. *Molecular Neurobiology*, **10**, 19–45.
35. Schubert, D., Jin, L.-W., Saitoh, T., *et al.* (1989) The regulation of amyloid beta protein precursor secretion and its modulatory role in cell adhesion. *Neuron*, **3**, 689–694.
36. Koo, E.H., Park, L. and Selkoe, D. (1993) Amyloid beta protein as a substrate interacts with extracellular matrix to promote neurite outgrowth. *Proceedings of the National Academy of Sciences, USA*, **90**, 4748–4752.
37. Moya, K.L., Benowitz, L.I., Schneider, G.E., *et al.* (1994) The amyloid precursor protein is developmentally regulated and correlated with synaptogenesis. *Developmental Biology*, **161**, 597–603.
38. Mattson, M., Barger, S.W., Cheng, B., *et al.* (1993) Beta amyloid precursor protein metabolites and loss of neuronal calcium homeostasis in Alzheimer's disease. *Trends in Neuroscience*, **16**, 409–414.
39. Muller, U., Cristina, N., Li, Z.-W., *et al.* (1994) Behavioral and anatomical deficits in mice homologous for a modified beta amyloid precursor protein gene. *Cell*, **79**, 755–765.
40. Smith-Swintosky, V.L., Pettigrew, L.C., Craddock, S.D., *et al.* (1994) Secreted forms of beta-amyloid precursor protein protect against ischemic brain injury. *Journal of Neurochemistry*, **63**, 781–784.
41. Mucke, L., Abraham, C.R., Ruppe, M.D., *et al.* (1995) Protection against HIV-1 gp120-induced brain damage by neuronal expression of human amyloid precursor protein. *Journal of Experimental Medicine*, **181**, 1551–1556.
42. Banati, R.B., Gehrmann, J., Lannes-Viera, J., *et al.* (1995) Inflammatory reaction in experimental encephalomyelitis (EAE) is accompanied by a microglial expression of the beta-amyloid precursor protein (APP). *Glia*, **14**, 209–215.
43. Mandelkow, E.-M., Schweers, O., Drewes, G., *et al.* (1996) Structure, microtubule interactions, and phosphorylation of tau protein. *Annals of the New York Academy of Sciences*, **777**, 96–106.
44. Gong, C.-X., Singh, T.J., Grundke-Iqbal, T.J., *et al.* (1994) Alzheimer disease abnormally phosphorylated tau is dephosphorylated by protein phosphatase-2B (calcineurin). *Journal of Neurochemistry*, **62**, 803–806.
45. Lee, V.M.-Y. (1996) Regulation of tau phosphorylation in Alzheimer's disease. *Annals of the New York Academy of Sciences*, **777**, 107–113.
46. Gong, X.-C., Grundke-Iqbal, I., Damuni, Z., *et al.* (1993). Dephosphorylation of microtubule associated protein tau by protein phosphatase 1 and 2C and its implication in Alzheimer disease. *FEBS Letters*, **341**, 94–98.
47. Tanaka, T., Iqbal, K., Trenkner, E., *et al.* (1995) Phosphatase inhibitors increase tau phosphorylation and induce cytotoxicity in SH-SY5Y neuroblastoma cells. *Society for Neuroscience*, **21**, 255 (abstract).
48. Strittmatter, W., Weisgraber, K., Huang, D., *et al.* (1993) Binding of human apolipoprotein E to synthetic amyloid beta peptide: isoform specific effects and implications for late onset Alzheimer's disease. *Procedings of the National Academy of Sciences, USA*, **90**, 8098–8102.
49. Sanan, D., Weisgraber, K., Russell, S., *et al.* (1994) Apolipoprotein E associates with β-amyloid peptide of Alzheimer's disease to form novel monofibrils. *Journal of Clinical Investigation*, **94**, 860–869.
50. Nathan, B., Bellosta, S., Sanan, D., *et al.* (1994) Differential effects of apolipoproteins E3 and E4 on neuronal growth *in vitro*. *Science*, **264**, 850–852.
51. Strittmatter, W.J., Weisgraber, K.H., Goedert, M., *et al.* (1994) Hypothesis: microtubule instability and paried helical filament formation in the Alzheimer disease brain are related to apolipoprotein E genotype. *Experimental Neurology*, **125**, 163–171.

52. Miyata, M. and Smith, J. (1996) Apolipoprotein E allele-specific antioxidant activity and effects on cytotoxicity by oxidative insults and B-amyloid peptides. *Nature Genetics*, **14**, 55–61.
53. Dunnett, S.B. and Fibiger, H.C. (1993) Role of forebrain cholinergic systems in learning and memory: relevance to the cognitive deficits of aging and AD dementia. *Progress in Brain Research*, **98**, 413–420.
54. Nitsch, R.M., Slack, R.J., Wurtman, J.H., *et al.* (1992) Release of Alzheimer amyloid precursor derivatives stimulated by activation of muscarinic acetylcholine receptors. *Science*, **258**, 304–307.
55. Kelly, J.F., Furukawa, K., Barger, S.W., *et al.* (1996) Amyloid beta-peptide disrupts carbacol-induced muscarinic cholinergic signal transduction in cortical neurons. *Procedings of the National Academy of Sciences, USA*, **93**, 6753–6758.
56. Whitehouse, P.J. (1993) Cholinergic therapy in dementia. *Acta Neurologica Scandinavica, suppl.*, **149**, 42–45.
57. Meyer, E.M., de Fiebre, C.M., Papke, R.L., *et al.* (1996) Cytoprotective actions of nicotinic receptor stimulation (abstract). *Fifth International Conference on Alzheimer's disease and Related Disorders*, Osaka, Japan.
58. Shimohama, S. (1996) Nicotinic agonists prevent neuronal cell death by glutamate and amyloid beta protein (abstract). *Fifth International Conference on Alzheimer's Disease and related disorders*, Osaka, Japan.
59. McGeer, P. and Rogers, J. (1992) Anti-inflammatory agents as a therapeutic approach to Alzheimer's disease. *Neurology*, **42**, 447–449.
60. Goodman, Y. and Mattson, M. (1994) Secreted forms of beta amyloid precursor protein protect hippocampal neurons against amyloid beta peptide induced oxidative injury. *Experimental Neurology*, **128**, 1–12.
61. Furuta, A., Price, D.L., Pardo, C.A., *et al.* (1995) Localization of superoxide dismutases in Alzheimer's disease and Down's syndrome neocortex and hippocampus. *American Journal of Pathology*, **146**, 357–367.
62. Lahiri, D.K. and Nall, C. (1995) Promoter activity of the gene incoding the beta-amyloid precursor protein is up-regulated by growth factors, phorbol ester, retinoic acid and interleukin-1. *Brain Research (Molecular Brain Research)*, **32**, 233–240.
63. Haring, R., Gurwitz, D., Barg, J., *et al.* (1995) NGF promotes amyloid precursor protein secretion via muscarinic receptor activation. *Biochemical and Biophysical Research Communications*, **213**, 15–23.
64. Bauman, K., Mandelkow, E.-M., Biernat, J., *et al.* (1993) Abnormal Alzheimer's like phosphorylation of tau protein by cyclin-dependent cdk2 and cdk5. *FEBS Letters*, **336**, 417–424.
65. Drewes, G., Mandelkow, E.-M., Bauman, K., *et al.* (1993) Dephosphorylation of tau protein and alzheimer paired helical filaments by calcineurin and phosphatase 2A. *FEBS Letters*, **336**, 425–432.
66. Biernat, J., Gustke, N., Drewes, G., *et al.* (1993) Phosphorylation of Ser262 strongly reduces binding of tau to microtubules: distinction between PHF-like immunoreactivity and microtubule binding. *Neuron*, **11**, 153–163.
67. Drewes, G., Trinczek, B., Illenberger, S., *et al.* (1995) Microtubule associated protein/microtubule affinity-regulating kinase (p110mark). A novel protein kinase that regulates tau-microtubule interactions and dynamic instability by phosphorylation at the Alzhiemer-specific site serine 262. *Journal of Biological Chemistry*, **270**, 7679–7688.
68. Iqbal, K. and Grundke-Iqbal, I. (1996) Molecular mechanism of Alzheimer's neurofibrillary degeneration and therapeutic intervention. *Annals of the New York Academy of Sciences*, **777**, 132–138.

69. De Fiebre, C.M., Meyer, E.M., Henry, J.C., *et al.* (1995) Characterization of a series of anabaseine-derived compounds reveals that the 3-(4)-dimethy-laminocinnamylidine derivative is a selective agonist at neuronal nicotinic alpha 7/125I-alpha-bungarotoxin receptor subtypes. *Molecular Pharmacology*, **47**, 164–171.

70. Rogers, J., Kirby, L.C., Hempelman, S.R., *et al.* (1993) Clinical trial of indomethacin in Alzheimer's disease. *Neurology*, **43**, 1609–1611.

71. Busciglio, J. and Yankner, B.A. (1995) Apoptosis and increased generation of reactive oxygen species in Down's syndrome neurons *in vitro*. *Nature*, **378**, 776–779.

72. Harris, M.E., Hensley, K., Butterfield, D.A., *et al.* (1995) Direct evidence of oxidative injury produced by the Alzheimer's beta-amyloid peptide (1–40) in cultured hippocampal neurons. *Experimental Neurology*, **131**, 193–202.

73. Brorson, J.R., Bindokas, V.P., Iwama, T., *et al.* (1995) The Ca^{2+} influx induced by beta-amyloid peptide 25–35 in cultured hippocampal neurons results from network excitation. *Journal of Neurobiology*, **26**, 325–338.

74. Dykens, J.A. (1994) Isolated cerebral and cerebellar mitochondria produce free radicals when exposed to elevated Ca^{2+} and Na^+: implications for neurodegeneration. *Journal of Neurochemistry*, **63**, 584–591.

75. Tollefson, G.D. (1990) Short-term effects of the calcium channel blocker nimodipine in the management of primary degenerative dementia. *Biological Psychiatry*, **27**, 1133–1142.

76. Scriabine, A. and van den Kerckhoff, W. (1988) Pharmacology of nimodipine. A review. *Annals of the New York Academy of Sciences*, **522**, 698–706.

77. Luiten, P.G., de Jong, G.I. and Schuurman, T. (1994) Cerebrovascular, neuronal, and behavioral effects of long-term Ca^{2+} channel blockade in aging normotensive and hypertensive rat strains. *Annals of the New York Academy of Sciences*, **747**, 431–451.

78. Kowalska, M. and Disterhoft, J.F. (1994) Relation of nimodipine dose and serum concentration to learning enhancement in aging rabbits. *Experimental Neurology*, **127**, 159–166.

6

Drugs for Alzheimer's disease

Lon S. Schneider and Pierre N. Tariot

INTRODUCTION

Alzheimer disease (AD) is the most common form of cognitive decline among older persons, afflicting 5% of people over age 65 years [1]. Except for rare early-onset familial cases, the causes are unknown. As the molecular mechanisms are clarified, treatments aimed at specific pathogenetic pathways will likely emerge. While awaiting further developments treatment of dementia is available for both the so-called core symptoms of cognitive deficit and the associated behavioral complications, including depression, agitation and psychosis [2]. In this chapter, we review currently available pharmacologic treatments for cognitive deficits, decline and new potential interventions that may affect underlying pathological processes in AD.

Before the 1980s, in general, medications were proposed for dementia treatment based on clinical experience or prevailing theories of dementia and aging. Examples of such earlier drugs included psychostimulants, vasodilators, ergoloids, nootropics and various medication 'cocktails'. Only one medication, Hydergine®, was approved on a worldwide basis for the ill-defined conditions of 'cerebral insufficiency' or 'cerebral deterioration' and, in the USA, explicitly for 'senile mental decline'.

The advent and acceptance of research-based diagnostic criteria for AD, the understanding of the underlying pathology, and mechanism-based pharmacological therapeutics provided the framework for clinical trials to exploit new treatment strategies. Although there are attempts to

Psychopharmacology of Cognitive and Psychiatric Disorders in the Elderly. Edited by David Wheatley and David Smith. Published in 1998 by Chapman and Hall, London.
ISBN 0 412 82470 1

gain recognition of functionally significant but mild cognitive loss such as benign senile forgetfulness, age-associated memory impairment (AAMI) or minimal cognitive impairment, the vagueness of the definitions and pathological correlates limit general acceptance. In this chapter, reference will be made to a number of diagnostic and severity measures used to record change. Chapter 7 should be consulted for descriptions of these.

CHOLINERGIC DRUGS

The prominent cholinergic dysfunction in AD has led to considerable focus on cholinergic restitutive strategies.

Precursor loading

Although many studies of the possible efficacy of cholinergic precursors in AD such as lecithin (phosphatidyl choline) have been conducted, results have not been clinically significant. Only 10 of 43 acetylcholine precursor trials reported any positive effect at all [3]. Trials in which lecithin was combined with the cholinesterase inhibitor tacrine did not reveal any added benefit.

Recently, however, cytidine diphosphate choline (CDP-choline), another acetylcholine precursor, has been assessed. Clinical trials have shown positive effects of CDP-choline in demented patients [4].

Cholinesterase inhibitors

The impetus for the development of cholinesterase inhibitors arose from early studies of physostigmine. Although improvements were modest, the drug was generally consistent in its memory effects when dosing was individualized [5]. Such dosage individualization has been a feature of multicenter trials of the cholinesterase inhibitors tacrine, velnacrine and sustained-release physostigmine using larger populations [6]. Physostigmine's very short duration of action (1–2 hours) and the brief durations of clinical trials (up to several weeks) have limited conclusions regarding its cognitive effects [for detailed citations see ref. 2].

Several cholinesterase inhibitors are available, will soon be available or are currently under phase III study for treatment of the cognitive symptoms (Table 6.1). They can be grouped into three classes according to their structure and mode of inhibition [7]:

(1) reversible tertiary and quaternary amines (e.g. tacrine, donepezil and galantamine);
(2) pseudo-irreversible carbamates (e.g. sustained-release physostigmine and ENA 713);
(3) irreversible, organophosphate inhibitors (e.g. metrifonate).

Table 6.1 Selected cholinergically active medications currently or recently under investigation for Alzheimer's disease

Cholinesterase inhibitors
Tacrine (Cognex®)
Velnacrine[a]
Donepezil (Aricept®, E2020)
ENA 713 (Exelon®)
Metrifonate
Sustained release physostigmine (Synapton)
Eptastigmine (heptyl-physostigmine)
Galantamine (Reminyl®)

Cholinergic agonists
Xanomeline
Milameline
AF 102B
SB 202026
ABT 418

Indirect cholinergic facilitators
Nicotine
DuP 996[a]
Ondansetron[a]

Other drugs with putative cholinergic effects
Acetyl-l-carnitine
Estrogens

[a] No longer under development for dementia

Tacrine was the first cholinesterase inhibitor to receive FDA marketing approval for the treatment of cognitive symptoms in AD, in September 1993, followed by donepezil in December 1996. ENA 713, physostigmine-SR and metrifonate have completed phase III studies and all will have filed applications for licensing in the US by the end of 1997.

Tacrine (Cognex®)

Tacrine is an acridine-based non-selective, reversible cholinesterase inhibitor with dose-dependent activity.

Pharmacology

Tacrine has a low but highly variable bioavailability when taken orally, but is rapidly absorbed with peak concentrations at about 1 hour. The short, but variable, elimination half-life of tacrine is prolonged with higher and multiple dosing (up to 3.6 hours) with a 4–6 hour duration of action. At least three metabolites result from hepatic transformation mainly by cytochrome CYP 1A2 hydroxylation and subsequent glucuronidation; the main metabolite is the (+)enantiomer 1-OH metabolite. Plasma levels are higher in women than in men and lower in cigarette smokers than in non-smokers, probably due to lower CYP 1A2 enzyme activity in women and its induction in smokers (Cognex package insert, Parke-Davis, Inc., © 1993).

Clinical studies

Following an initial case series that claimed dramatic improvements [8], smaller crossover studies showed less impressive results [for detailed reviews see refs 9, 10]. Larger scale studies tended to clarify tacrine's efficacy (Table 6.2) [11–16]. Results overall show statistically significant differences in favor of tacrine on various cognitive, functional, caregiver and clinician ratings. Some outcome measures did not show statistically significant differences in these trials and a substantial number of patients were discontinued because of transaminase elevations above usually three times the upper limit of normal (see below).

Two studies were considered for licensing purposes in the USA, and elsewhere. In a two-stage, 12-week parallel-group trial comparing 80, 40 and 20 mg/day of tacrine with placebo [12], significant differences in favor of tacrine were observed on the ADAS cognitive subscale outcome criterion, the CGIC and a caregiver-rated change score in 77 patients treated with 80 mg/day during the last 6 weeks of the 12-week trial.

The most comprehensive efficacy trial [14] was a 30-week-long parallel-group study involving 663 patients who were randomized to three dosage treatments or placebo. The daily dosage of tacrine was increased at six-week intervals by 40 mg per day. Statistically significant treatment effects were observed for the 120 and 160 mg per day groups at 30 weeks on both the ADAS-cog and a clinician interview-based impression of change although there was a very high dropout rate in the tacrine group because of excessive transaminase elevations.

Dosing

The FDA-approved dosing regimen is an artifact of the forced titration study design, recommending that tacrine be started at 10 mg q.i.d. and maintained for six weeks. The dose of tacrine should then be increased to 20 mg q.i.d. providing there is no intolerance or increase in transaminase levels above three times the upper limit of normal. After six weeks, dosage should be increased to 30 mg q.i.d., again with weekly monitoring. And then, if tolerated, to 40 mg q.i.d. for the next six weeks. During this time serum transaminase levels are monitored biweekly. Effective doses of tacrine are above 120 mg per day.

Table 6.2 Larger randomized placebo-controlled clinical trials of tacrine (with or without lecithin) lasting 12 weeks or more

Study	Sample size (randomized/ analyzed)[a]	Duration[b]	Dose[c]	Design	Results/comments
Eagger et al. (1991) [11]	89 or 64	13 weeks	120 mg Lecithin, 10.8 g	2-period crossover trial with 4-week washout. Dose was titrated during first week each period.	Tacrine plus lecithin was compared with lecithin. Analyzed as a 13-week parallel-group trial (n=89). Significant results on the MMSE and the Abbreviated Mental Test Score (AMTS).
Farlow et al. (1992) [12]	468/273	12 weeks	80 mg/d 40 mg 20 mg	Parallel-group 12-week, 2-stage, dose escalation, 3 treatment groups plus placebo	77 patients treated with 80 mg/day at 12 weeks and 77 placebo patients. Significant improvement on ADAS-Cog. CGIC and caregiver's CGIC. Multisite study.
Wilcock et al. (1993) [13]	85/41	12 weeks	< 60–120 mg	2-period crossover, with 4-week washout	Trend for MMSE (P=0.07) for 1st period effect and crossover analysis (P=0.13) and for a functional scale (P=0.09)
Knapp et al. (1994) [14]	663/286	30 weeks	160 mg/d 120 mg 80 mg	Parallel-group, ascending dose, 3 treatment groups plus placebo	Significant dose-trend effects favoring tacrine on the ADAS-Cog, CIBI, MMSE, a severity scale and a caregiver-CGIC.
Maltby et al. (1994) [15]	41/32	9 months	54 mg/d < 80 mg Lecithin, 10.8 g	Parallel-group	No significant differences on 21 of 22 outcome tests. All received doses of less than 80 mg/d of tacrine.
Wood et al. (1994) [16]	154/131	12 weeks	70 mg/d[e]	Parallel-group, flexible dosage	Significant improvement on clinicians' and relatives' global ratings; no significant improvement on MMSE or 3 other scales. Less than one-half of patients received doses of 80 mg/d or more of tacrine

ADAS; Alzheimer Disease Assessment Scale; Cog: cognitive subscale; CIBI; Clinician's Interview-Based Impression of Change; CGIC: Clinician's Global Impression of Change; MMSE: Mini-mental State Examination.

[a]Sample size analyzed at end of study. Numbers are approximate since they may vary within study depending on the particular outcome instrument. The number of patients who entered these trials was usually considerably greater.

[b]Duration of treatment period used for efficacy analysis; does not include pre-randomization dose-titration periods. In most trials, there was a 6-week dose-finding phase and a 2-week placebo phase before the efficacy segment.

[c]Median, average, maximum, or range of daily dose of efficacy evaluation.

[d]Dosages indicated are those at end of trial.

[e]All but 3 patients received doses < 80 mg/d

Adverse effects

Adverse reactions include the expected cholinergic effects and, additionally, asymptomatic serum transaminase elevation from hepatotoxic drug metabolism. Peripheral cholinergic effects, such as nausea, vomiting, diarrhea, dyspepsia or appetite loss, occur in 10–20% (Cognex package insert, Warner-Lambert Co., 1993). In general, dose-related side-effects are mild, short-lived and can usually be managed by dosage modification or reducing the dosage temporarily as tolerance appears to develop.

The most frequent adverse event associated with tacrine is asymptomatic, reversible, direct hepatocellular injury characterized by elevations in serum aminotransferases. Elevations above three times the upper limit of normal occur in approximately 30% of patients, tend to occur between the fifth and seventh week of treatment, and tend to be transient, returning to normal over several weeks. Over 90% of all transaminase elevations occur within 12 weeks of initiating treatment. If the level is less than five times the upper limit of normal then the dosage should be reduced by 40 mg a day until the transaminases fall. If the dose is above five times the upper limit of normal than medication should be stopped until levels return to normal limits. At that point patients may be rechallenged (see the package insert for full prescribing information).

Velnacrine

Velnacrine is a racemic mixture of 1-hydroxytacrine with similar magnitude and quality of clinical effects (Table 6.3) and side-effects to tacrine including reversible asymptomatic serum transaminase elevations similar in incidence to tacrine, but with the additional evidence of depressed leukocyte counts. The clinical development of velnacrine was discontinued once tacrine was approved. Its main significance is as a non-specific cholinesterase inhibitor that shows similar therapeutic effects to others [17].

Sustained-release physostigmine salicylate (Synapton®)

Unpublished results from this relatively new, longer-acting controlled-release formulation of physostigmine from phase III trials indicate efficacy on both cognitive and clinicians' interview-based ratings, with the expected peripheral cholinergic side-effects. A new drug application may be filed in the US by late 1997.

Second-generation cholinesterase inhibitors

The newer cholinesterase inhibitors suggest the advantages of longer action, differing selectivities of acetylcholinesterase inhibition, and of fewer, more predictable side effects. Data from phase II and III trials sug-

Table 6.3 Key phase II or III randomized placebo-controlled parallel-group clinical trials of cholinesterase inhibitors in Alzheimer's disease

Drug	Dosage arms (mg)	Size[a]	Duration[b] (wks)	Completers[1]	Adverse events	Outcome (drug-placebo difference) ADASc	CGIC (% improved)	Results/comments
Tacrine[12]	20 q.i.d. 10 q.i.d.	468/273	12	48%	Elevated ALTs, nausea and/or vomiting, diarrhea, anorexia, dyspepsia, abdominal pain	3.8	0.5	25% of tacrine-treated patients were withdrawn because of ALTs > 3 × ULN
Tacrine[14]	40 q.i.d. 30 q.i.d. 20 q.i.d.	663/653/263	30	42% 29% dropped out b/o ALT elevations	Elevated ALTs, nausea and/or vomiting, diarrhea, anorexia, dyspepsia, abdominal pain	2.2 5.3	0.2 23% vs 17% 0.5 42% vs 18%	ITT analysis above; completer analysis below. 28% were withdrawn because of ALT elevations > 3 × ULN
Velnacrine[17]	75 t.i.d. 50 t.i.d.	449/280	24	62%	Elevated ALTs, diarrhea, vomiting, anorexia. Possible leukopenia	2.4	.30	No longer being developed. LOCF analysis. 26% of tacrine-treated patients were withdrawn because of ALT elevations > 5 × ULN
Donepezil (package insert)	10 q.d. 5 q.d.	468	12		Nausea, vomiting, diarrhea, fatigue, muscle cramps	3.0	0.38 39% vs 18%	ITT analysis
Donepezil (package insert)	10 q.d. 5 q.d.	473	24	68%	Nausea, vomiting, diarrhea, fatigue, muscle cramps	3.1	0.39 25% vs 12%	ITT analysis
ENA 713[19]	6–12 q.d. 1–4 q.d.	699	26	65%	Nausea, vomiting, diarrhea, anorexia	4.6	0.29 22% vs 15%	ITT analysis. Other studies pending.
Metrifonate (1997)	30–60 mg	408	25	79%	Diarrhea, leg cramps, rhinitis, decreased HR	2.8	0.28	ITT analysis. Other studies pending

Figures are only approximate as it is not always clear what the denominator was and different standards were used among trials completers. Adverse events listed generally those occurring significantly more often than placebo at the highest dose. Outcome effect sizes are drug-placebo differences and are based on the highest dose used in the trial. All effects listed are statistically significant at the P < 0.05 level, two-tailed. Differences in outcome are not comparable among studies especially on clinicians' global' ratings and should be used as a guide only, since actual differences depend on statistics all model, type of analysis, and are not performed consistently from study to study. Trials were done at different times, with different criteria and have varying placebo effects and therefore cannot be compared.

1 Completers reported from the highest dose in each study.

Abbreviations

ALTs: alanine aminotransferase;

ITT: intent-to-treat analysis

LOCF: last observation carried forward analysis

ULN: upper limit of normal

[a] Approximate sample number and randomized/number analyzed.

[b] Duration of randomized placebo-controlled treatment period.

gest efficacy comparable to that of tacrine for many of these newer compounds, with a similar frequency of cholinergic effects but no significant elevation of serum tranaminases.

Donepezil (E2020, Aricept®)

Donepezil (Aricept®, Eisai/Pfizer, formerly E2020), is a piperidine-based, reversible cholinesterase inhibitor that has dose-dependent activity, showing greater selectivity for acetylcholinesterase than some other cholinesterases and a longer duration of cholinesterase inhibition than tacrine, ENA 713 or physostigmine-SR [18]. The drug received approval for marketing in the US by the FDA in November 1996 and in the UK in April 1997.

Pharmacology

It is characterized by linear pharmacokinetics at therapeutic doses with a slow clearance and a 70-hour elimination half-life allowing steady state to be achieved in 12–14 days. The bioavailability of donepezil approaches 100% with peak concentrations at three hours. The drug is extensively bound to plasma proteins. It is both excreted unchanged in the urine and extensively metabolized to active and inactive metabolites in the liver by CYP 2D6 and 3A4, conjugated and excreted. Although there is little experience with donepezil-drug interactions, it follows that inhibitors of 3A4 and 2D6 may inhibit the metabolism of donepezil and that inducers of the enzymes could decrease plasma levels. However, plasma levels are sufficiently low so that interactions may not be significant.

Clinical studies

There have been three published placebo-controlled trials, one phase II, examining doses up to 5 mg/day [18], and two phase III trials examining doses of 5 and 10 mg/day for 12 and 24 weeks, respectively. Results of the latter studies showed statistically significant benefit in both subscales and clinicians' rated change scale (Table 6.3 and package insert).

In the 24-week study 473 patients were randomized to receive doses of placebo or donepezil (5 mg q.d. or 10 mg q.d.). At the end of 24 weeks, patients in each treatment group showed significant differences from placebo on the ADAS-cog, the neuropsychological outcome measure and on the CGIC measure. Similarly, in the 12-week study there were significant differences on the ADAS-cog and the CGIC between donepezil and placebo. There is a trend toward a greater effect of 10 mg/day throughout the course of treatment but not at the end of 24 weeks. In both studies, following discontinuation of donepezil, the cognitive scores approached that of the placebo group after three to six weeks.

Dosing

Patients should be started on 5 mg/day for two to four weeks, and if toler-ated raised to 10 mg/day. The efficacy or appropriateness of higher doses has not been established.

Adverse effects

In the placebo-controlled trials patients who received 5 mgd withdrew at the same rate as placebo-treated patients (about 15–20%), whereas approximately twice as many patients who received 10 mg withdrew from the trials largely due to cholinergic side effects. Most common adverse events included nausea, diarrhea, vomiting, muscle cramps, fatigue, anorexia and insomnia. Symptoms are generally of mild intensity and short-lived, tending to resolve with continuing treatment and to be related to the rate at which dosages are increased; however, nausea, diar-rhea or vomiting together were responsible for approximately 8–9% of patients who withdrew at 10 mg per day.

ENA 713 (Exelon®)

ENA 713 (Sandoz) is a pseudo-irreversible carbamate-selective acetyl-cholinesterase subtypes inhibitor. It is characterized by its selective inacti-vation of acetylcholinesterase and is not metabolized by the hepatic microsome system [19]. Rather, after binding to acetylcholinesterase the carbamate portion of the molecule is slowly hydrolyzed, conjugated to a sulphate and excreted. Its duration of actylcholinesterase inhibition is approximately 10 hours.

Four six-month long trials have been completed involving 10 countries and 2800. Preliminary results, presented at various meetings in 1996 and 1997, from the flexible-dose range USA study indicate that doses of 6–12 mg per day were associated with improvements on the ADASc, clinicians, global rating and activity of daily living (ADLs). About 65% of patients completed the six month studies at higher doses compared to 85% on placebo and there was dose-dependent activity, with higher doses gener-ally associated with greater improvement and cholinergic effects. A new drug application was filed in April 1997. FDA approval is anticipated by early 1998.

Metrifonate

Widely used in the past as an anti-schistosomiasis agent, metrifonate is an organophosphorus prodrug that does not inhibit cholinesterase itself but is metabolized to the long-acting cholinesterase inhibitor, dichlorvos (2,2 dimethyl dichlorovinyl phosphate). The RBC cholinesterase inhibi-tion half-life is nearly two months, meaning that the effect will be chronic. Phase II dosing trials over 12 weeks have shown significant effects on both the ADAS cognitive scale and global scales, with the typical expected cholinergic symptoms [20]. One phase III six-month study has reported showing significant improvements in cognition and global ratings [21]. Results of other phase III studies are pending. A new drug application will be filed in the US by January 1998.

Eptastigmine

Eptastigmine (heptylphysostigmine, Mediolanum) is a hydrophobic derivative of physostigmine with a duration of action of six to eight hours. Effective doses may range from 30 to 60 mg per day with the expected cholinergic side effects. There are reports of occasional reversible decreases in neutrophil count. A recent phase III trial involving 26 centers in Italy and the USA and 320 patients compared two doses of eptastigmine with placebo over 25 weeks and demonstrated significant efficacy on the ADAS-cog [22].

Galantamine

Galantamine is a competitive reversible cholinesterase inhibitor and nicotinic receptor modulator with relatively greater selectivity for acetylcholinesterase than other cholinesterases, that was originally isolated from the snowdrop flower. It has a duration of action of approximately 10 hours; daily doses may range from 16 to 32 mg. Phase III trials are ongoing.

Muscarinic and nicotinic agonists

The observations in AD that postsynaptic M_1 cholinergic receptors are relatively intact and presynaptic M_2 cholinergic receptors are decreased provide a rationale for direct cholinergic agonists. Early pilot trials with bethanechol, oxotremorine, pilocarpine, RS-86, and arecoline did not demonstrate meaningful efficacy and were associated with significant cholinergic side effects. Intracerebroventricular administration of bethanechol resulted in small yet statistically significant improvement on the MMSE but there is substantial risk from the surgical procedures [for references, see ref 2].

Other cholinergic agonists with relatively low toxicity and with relatively greater affinity for M_1 receptors are currently being tested in clinical trials and may be more promising. Examples of such agents include xanomeline, milameline, AF102B and SB202026. AF102B and SB202026 are partial agonists that are functionally selective for M_1 muscarinic receptors with lower affinity for other muscarinic receptors. Milameline appears to be non-selective. A dose-ranging study of AF102B in escalating doses of 20, 40, 60 mg t.i.d. over 10 weeks suggested that higher doses were associated with improved word recognition [23].

The use of transdermal nicotine and partial nicotinic agonists such as ABT 418 may enhance presynaptic release of acetylcholine and represent other potential therapeutics. Clinical trials are planned or underway with these agents.

DuP 996 (linopirdine) and ondansetron, a 5-HT$_3$ antagonist, are two additional indirect presynaptic releasers of acetylcholine but neither demonstrated efficacy.

LONG-TERM EFFECTS OF CHOLINERGIC AGENTS

Cholinergic stimulation *in vitro* may have profound long-term effects on neuronal function and survival. For example, stimulation of M$_1$ receptors by AF102B enhances secretion of amyloid precursor protein derivatives and decreases tau phosphorylation and, therefore, may be of value in delaying the progression of AD.

Early small-scale uncontrolled studies suggest that long-term use of physostigmine may retard cognitive deterioration, even in patients who fail to improve following acute doses [24–27]. Similarly, relative preservation of cognitive function and nicotinic binding was reported with tacrine [28, 29] and metrifonate [20]. Recently, it was reported in a cohort study that the chronic use of higher doses of tacrine (> 120–160 mg/day) over the course of approximately two years was associated with a delay in nursing home placement of approximately 400 days and an overall lesser liklihood of placement (RR = 0.37) [30].

FACTORS INVOLVED IN RESPONSE TO CHOLINESTERASE INHIBITORS

In view of overall limitations in treatment response, it would be desirable to determine the predictors of maximum beneficial response. Although AD is a clinically and biologically heterogeneous illness, published trials tend to select patients who are relatively homogeneous and provide limited information on heterogeneous characteristics [for detailed references see ref. 31].

As the vast majority of patients treated with cholinesterase inhibitors have been of European descent, there is insufficient information about possible ethnic differences in response.

Age

The contribution of age to treatment response is difficult to assess as clinical trials have used restricted age ranges with very few subjects under age 65 or over 85 years. In one report [32], increasing age was correlated with metabolite plasma levels ($r = 0.35$ to 0.47), plasma levels were significantly correlated with clinical response ($r = 0.23$ to 0.32), but age itself was not correlated with response.

Sex

Although sex is not strongly associated with clinical response, women receiving estrogen replacement therapy (ERT) and those with a non-ApoE 4 genotype were reported to have a larger magnitude of response when treated with tacrine than women not receiving ERT (M.R. Farlow *et al.*, unpublished results) [33].

Dementia severity

In small studies patients with earlier phases or less cognitive impairment had greater improvements in MMSE on tacrine therapy [34,35]. In a re-analysis of a multicenter trial of tacrine with dosage of 160 mg per day [14], although similar levels of improvement were seen from baseline whether the patients were in a mild or moderate stage, deterioration from baseline in the placebo group was much greater in patients with moderate illness. Therefore the treatment effects of tacrine were substantially greater in patients with moderate stage illness [36].

The insensitivity of the ADAS-cog to change at the early stages makes it difficult to rule out a greater effect in very early stages. Early demented and highly educated patients perform very well on the cognitive rating scales, making it difficult to evidence numerical improvement over the three to six months of the study. The question of whether dementia severity predicts response to cholinesterase inhibitors remains open.

Behavioral symptoms

Baseline impairments in activities do not predict response per se [26] but a secondary analysis of the tacrine data suggested that patients with delusions responded better than those without [37].

Cognitive features

Early studies with physostigmine showed modest short-term improvements areas such as selective reminding, delayed recall, picture recognition, finger tapping and category generation. Analyses on subscales of the ADAS in multicenter tacrine trials reveal significance in word recall, object naming, language and word finding [12], but no significant pattern of response on factor analyses [38]. In one trial, however, tacrine treatment was more associated with improvement in attention [39] and dysphasia prior to treatment was associated with a poorer outcome [11].

Dementia subtype

Clinical characteristics of diffuse Lewy body disease are similar to AD, but include also a fluctuating cognitive impairment, with episodic confusion and lucid intervals associated with hallucinations and extrapyramidal findings and the decrease in choline acetyltransferase is more pronounced than in AD without Lewy bodies [40]. Patients with autopsy-confirmed AD and diffuse Lewy body disease were reported to be marked responders to tacrine but confirming studies are needed [29,41].

Apolipoprotein E profile

In light of observations that AD patients with the apolipoprotein E4 allele have both an increased risk for the illness and possibly a more rapid course [42], results from the 30-week tacrine trial show that women not carrying the apoE4 allele had a greater treatment effect (drug-placebo difference) than men not carrying an apoE4 allele or either men or women with an apoE4 allele (M.R. Farlow, unpublished results).

Dosage and plasma levels

Overall, cholinesterase inhibitor clinical studies have consistently shown a dose-response effect [18,32,43] and with higher doses associated with increased RBC cholinesterase inhibition, and with improved performance on cognitive function.

SUMMARY OF CHOLINERGIC THERAPIES

Despite the absence of direct comparisons, evidence so far suggests that cholinesterase inhibitors have roughly similar acute efficacy and a variable frequency of mild cholinergic side effects, both generally dependent on dose. (Reversible elevations of hepatic transaminases uniquely distinguish tacrine and are not a property of cholinesterase inhibitors or of dose.) The newer cholinesterase inhibitors offer the promise of less frequent dosing, greater patient acceptance and will likely prove to be more frequently used in the community than tacrine. Yet it is unlikely that patients will respond differently to individual cholinesterase inhibition and that individualization of drug and dosage will be important for maximal response.

The magnitude of improvement with cholinesterase inhibitors has been modest overall, but the proportion of patients who respond clinically under the best of conditions has ranged between 20% and 50% in trials depending on the exact definition for response. Age, sex and ethnicity are not clinically meaningful predictors of response to cholinesterase inhibitors, although women receiving ERT or who do not have an apoE4 allele *may* respond somewhat better to tacrine. Adequate dosages and plasma levels appear to be most important to therapeutic response, suggesting the first obvious strategy to enhance response. These observations need to be verified, but there is no published basis to withhold a cholinergic medication from an AD patient because he or she is deemed to have a 'poor' probability of responding, or is too mildly or severely impaired.

Cholinergic agonists are still relatively early in their development, but if successful, may represent an alternative or addition to cholinesterase inhibitors. Appropriately designed clinical trials are needed to assess for disease-modifying effects.

OTHER NEUROTRANSMITTER-BASED APPROACHES

Central catecholaminergic disturbances in AD provide a rationale for pharmacological enhancement and strategies are analogous to those used with cholinergic agents, i.e. precursor loading, degradative enzyme inhibition and agonist use. Studies of tryptophan, tyrosine, l-dopa and such agonists as clonidine, guanefacine, amantadine, bromocriptine and memantine have failed to demonstrate efficacy.

By contrast, monoamine oxidase (MAO) inhibitors have demonstrated some acute effects. Selegiline (l-deprenyl, Eldepryl®) is a MAO inhibitor with relatively selective inhibition of MAO type B [44]. At 5–10 mg daily, selegiline may increase central levels of dopamine and other neurotransmitters without an effect on norepinephrine levels. Studies of behavioral effects on patients with dementia indicate that selegiline may improve cooperativeness, anxiety, depression and agitation [45]. Open label studies show cognitive effects in AD, but an adequate efficacy trial has not been completed (see below) [for detailed references see ref. 44].

Citalopram, a serotonin uptake inhibitor, has demonstrated efficacy for behavioral symptoms [46], whereas other serotonin-acting compounds have had no significant effects on behavior or cognition, including zimelidine, tryptophan, alapracolate and m-chlorphenylpiperazine [for more complete references see ref. 2].

Excitatory amino acids

The N-methyl-D-aspartate (NMDA) receptor, a glutamate receptor subtype, is involved in memory function. When the excitatory amino acid glutamate stimulates the receptor, long-term potentiation of neuronal activity basic to memory formation occurs [47]. In AD, cerebral cortical and hippocampal NMDA receptors are decreased. Several drugs that could improve memory by regulating NMDA receptor transmission are now being developed. Memantine (1-amino-3,5-dimethyladamantane), another NMDA antagonist, is also under investigation although an initial study showed no effect.

Excitatory amino acids such as glutamate and aspartate may both enhance cognitive function and be neurotoxic. Stimulation of the glutamate receptor subtype of the NMDA receptor may improve memory. Excessive stimulation of glutamate receptors also is associated with brain injury. Studies using D-cycloserine and milacemide for AD have been without success.

Peptides

Several neuropeptide neurotransmitter systems are known to be disrupted in AD, including somatostatin, corticotrophin-releasing factor, neuropeptide Y and substance P. Neuropeptides are of potential interest as they modulate other neurotransmitter systems that may be dysregulated in AD.

Arginine vasopressin and several of its analogues led to modest improvements in behavior, possibly related to improved energy and mood, with no or very mild improvement in memory. The same is true of adrenocorticotrophic hormone agonists which appear to affect mood and behavior without clear memory or cognitive effects. A somatostatin analogue was administered to a small group of AD patients without cognitive effect. Although TRH had been shown to have possible beneficial cognitive effects in two small pilot studies, studies of TRH analogues have been negative.

Endogenous opiates may function as peptide neurotransmitters as well. Although naloxone, an opiate receptor antagonist, was initially reported to improve cognitive function in AD, these findings were not confirmed by subsequent studies or with the mixed agonist-antagonist, naltrexone.

OTHER APPROACHES DIRECTED AT PUTATIVE PATHOLOGICAL MECHANISMS

There are several convergent processes involved with the neuronal degeneration of AD, including oxidative damage, immunological and inflammatory responses, and the release of auto-destructive enzymes (Chapter 7). Some of these may not be specific to AD but rather may be associated with aging and neuronal death in general. These targeted interventions may be effective in modifying illness course.

Antioxidants

The therapeutic effects of selegiline (l-deprenyl) have been linked to its antioxidant and neuroprotective properties, as well as to enhancement of neurotransmitters [48]. Oxidative deamination of endogenous mono-amines by MAO results in the formation of toxic byproducts such as hydrogen peroxide, hydroxyl radicals and superoxides [49]. Oxidation of some monoamines by MAO, including dopamine, can produce neurotoxins such as 6-hydroxydopamine and quinone.

Thus, one rationale for possible beneficial effects of selegiline over the long term is a putative reduction of free radicals and neurotoxins resulting from inhibition of MAO-B activity. Indeed, *in vitro* data indicate that selegiline reduces the oxidative stress associated with catabolism of dopamine [49]. If this theoretical rationale is borne out, selegiline may conceivably have a preventative role in the development of neurodegenerative disorders or even normal aging. Increased survival has been reported in rodents treated with selegiline although data are not available for humans [50].

Recent longer term studies with selegiline have yielded mixed results but sample sizes were relatively small; the outcome effect sizes were large enough to suggest that a significant effect may have been observed with a larger sample size. A completed multicenter trial assessing the value of selegiline (5 mg b.i.d.) and vitamin E (dl-α-tocopherol, 1000 IU b.i.d.) in prolonging time to nursing home placement and other endpoints found that either drug alone prolonged time to reach endpoint but that the combination was less effective [51].

Other antioxidants

Antioxidant vitamins such as dl-α-tocopherol, ascorbic acid and coenzyme Q may also have efficacy in AD. Idebonone, an analogue of coenzyme Q, was effective at improving cognitive and global functioning in two recently reported trials [52].

Anti-inflammatories

Patients with rheumatoid arthritis who receive chronic anti-inflammatory treatment have a reduced risk for AD compared with controls without rheumatoid arthritis [53] and twins who used anti-inflammatory medications had lesser risk for AD than their co-twins [54]. A placebo-controlled trial of indomethacin supports a potential role for anti-inflammatory drugs [55]. A US National Institute of Aging Consortium is currently conducting a one-year, placebo-controlled trial of low-dose prednisone (10 mg) [56]. Because of gastrointestinal and other potential adverse effects from anti-inflammatory agents, newer anti-inflammatories may offer promise (e.g. cyclo-oxygenase-2 inhibitors) but require testing.

Anti-amyloid strategies

JTP-4819 is an inhibitor of prolyl endopeptidase, a protease that cleaves Aβ from amyloid precursor protein, and thus it may decrease the formation of Aβ (Chapter 7). In addition, it inhibits the degradation or enhances the function of several neuropeptides associated with memory and increases acetylcholine release. Early trials for dosing, efficacy and safety are ongoing. Its main significance is as a first drug intended to affect Aβ production.

Calcium channel blockers

As intracellular free calcium activates various destructive enzymes (e.g. proteases, endonucleases, phospholipases) and may mediate neuronal death from aging and AD, blocking intracellular free calcium could retard neuronal death and slow disease progression. One trial of nimodipine found that patients in the low-dose group (30 mg t.i.d.) had less memory deterioration after 12 weeks of treatment than those receiving placebo or high dose nimodipine (60 mg t.i.d.) [57], and another reported significant cognitive effects for nimodipine when compared with Hydergine® or placebo [58]. Nimodipine is marketed as a cognitive-enhancing agent and for stroke in Europe.

Neurotrophic factors

Nerve growth factor (NGF), a cholinergic trophic factor, counteracts cholinergic atrophy in the nucleus basalis although no direct evidence supports an NGF involvement in AD pathogenesis. Administering NGF to humans with AD may slow the rate of cholinergic neuronal degeneration, enhance neuronal function and thus improve behaviors caused by cholinergic deficits [59]. An intraventricular catheter and pump or carrier molecules are necessary for the administration of NGF as it does not cross the blood–brain barrier. European trials of intrathecal NGF demonstrated limited success [60]. Other proposed strategies include alkaloid-like molecules that cross the blood–brain barrier and may potentiate NGF activity, intraparenchymal administration, tissue transplant or injection of genetically modified cells.

Estrogens

Estrogens also may improve cognitive function through cholinergic neuroprotective and neurotrophic effects. For example, estradiol replacement enhances learning in ovariectomized rats; it also decreases choline uptake and ChAT levels resulting from ovariectomy.

Observations of an inverse relation between estrogen replacement therapy (ERT) exposure and a diagnosis of dementia as recorded on death certificates were followed by a cohort study of 470 women in the Baltimore Longitudinal Study. Subjects were followed for 16 years and women who received ERT showed a 54% reduction in risk for AD. Another recent report included approximately 1124 elderly women over a five-year period, observing that women who received ERT for a decade or more showed a 30–40% reduction in the risk of developing AD. These studies, however, require empirical verification. Five preliminary trials have reported estradiol, estrone and conjugated estrogens to enhance cognitive function in AD. Moreover, cognitive enhancing effects on verbal memory have been demonstrated in studies of cognitively intact post-menopausal women. Most post-menopausal women, however, decide not to take ERT and thus spend much of their later years in an estrogen-deficient state, when their risk for AD is highest. An analysis of the 30-week tacrine trial indicated that women receiving ERT (generally Premarin at a median dose of 0.625 mg/day) had a greater response to tacrine than those not on ERT [33]. Ongoing clinical trials are assessing whether conjugated estrogens (Premarin) influence cognitive functioning in women with AD or whether they delay AD onset (National Institute of Health Women's Health Initiative).

In summary, a possible role for ERT appears promising but there is a lack of large scale placebo-controlled clinical trials [for review and references see ref. 61].

OTHER APPROACHES

Propentofylline

Propentofylline is a xanthine derivative which acts both as an inhibitor of adenosine uptake and as a phosphodiesterase inhibitor. Increased intrasynaptic adenosine may increase adenosine receptor stimulation, reducing excitatory amino acid transmission. In addition, it may stimulate NGF and inhibit free radical production [62]. Clinical trials in patients with AD and vascular dementia over six and 12 months showed improvement in cognitive and global function compared to placebo [63]. Phase III trials are ongoing.

Acetyl-l-carnitine

Acetyl-l-carnitine has a structure similar to acetylcholine, promotes acetylcholine synthesis by providing acetyl groups, enhances high-affinity uptake of choline, has cholinomimetic effects on cholinergic receptors and may exert a 'neuroprotective' effect. Although it showed significant effects in earlier placebo-controlled trials of patients with unclear dementia criteria, a one-year multicenter trial in AD showed no overall effects, but an attenuation of cognitive worsening in patients under the age of 65 years (Thal *et al.*, unpublished results). Therefore, this agent is currently undergoing a confirmatory trial in younger patients with AD.

Membrane enhancers

Gangliosides, components of cell membranes with neurotrophic activity and possible protective effects against ischemia, are markedly diminished in cholinergically innervated areas of AD brains. Ganglioside GM-1, which increases neuronal responsiveness to neurotrophic factors and enhances neuronal plasticity and repair, has beneficial effects in the treatment of stroke. Phosphatidylserine, a naturally occurring phospholipid, can alter membrane fluidity. Clinical results suggested efficacy for severely impaired compared with less impaired AD patients.

Chelators

Although evidence is conflicting, some epidemiological studies suggest that aluminum exposure contributes to increased risk for AD pathogenesis. In addition, other metals such as iron and zinc have been proposed as risk factors for AD, but the mechanism by which the metals may exert their effects is unclear. Aluminum, iron and zinc tend to promote Aβ aggregation *in vitro*, suggesting that high concentrations of certain metals may contribute to the pathogenetic process in AD. The observations with aluminum led to trials of chelating agents, one of which, with EDTA, had no effect and the other, with desferrioxamine, was reported to slow disease progression, although this observation has not been corroborated (for references see ref. 2].

HYDERGINE

Hydergine®, a combination of four dihydro derivatives of ergotoxine, is the longest used putative cognitive enhancing drug and one of the most commonly prescribed drugs worldwide, although not in the USA. It is currently used primarily for patients with dementia or age-associated cognitive symptoms. The FDA approved Hydergine for 'idiopathic decline in mental capacity'. Numerous randomized, double-blinded, placebo-controlled clinical trials in a variety of elderly patient populations generally yielded effects favoring Hydergine although some trials were conflicting. However, these studies are difficult to interpret because of methodological limitations, including inadequately diagnosed and clinically heterogeneous subjects, the over-reliance on a particular outcome instrument, the focus on the improvement of individual behavioral symptoms, a general lack of attention to cognitive outcome and variable doses and study durations [for references see ref. 64]. Therefore, the clinical meaning of the results is unclear, although a recent meta-analysis suggested that Hydergine's effects may be greater in vascular dementia [65].

Nicergoline is another ergoloid derivative available in Europe. This drug has shown significant effects on orientation and attention [65].

NOOTROPICS

The nootropics are a drug class with diverse actions, structurally related to piracetam, which may improve memory and learning. In addition to piracetam, they include oxiracetam, pramiractam, aniracetam, CI 933 and BMY 21502. Nootropics may protect the CNS from potential damage due to hypoxia and may also enhance the CNS microcirculation through reductions of platelet activity and adherence of red blood cells to vessel walls. An anti-dementia mechanism has not been established and controlled trials yield mixed results. Clinical trials in AD have produced conflicting results but generally in studies using patients with dementias similar to AD, the magnitude of cognitive effects is comparable to other medications [66]. They are, however, marketed for dementia and cognitive impairment in many countries.

SUMMARY

Current treatment options licenced in many countries include the cholinesterase inhibitors tacrine, donepezil and ENA 713; sustained-release physostigmine and metrifonate may be available soon. Other drugs that affect the cholinergic system are in development. Some antioxidants, anti-inflammatories and estrogens are marketed worldwide, not indicated for dementia, but their efficacy is still not proven. Although no currently available anti-dementia treatment has been shown to have dramatic effects in improving the cognitive impairments of AD there may be improvements that are nonetheless clinically meaningful and considerable. Worldwide research and development efforts offer promise of more effective approaches in the future.

REFERENCES

1. Brayne, C., Gill, C., Huppert, F.A., *et al.* Incidence of clinically diagnosed subtypes of dementia in an elderly population. Cambridge Project for Later Life. *Br J Psychiatry* **167**, 255–262, 1995.
2. Schneider, L.S. and Tariot, P.N. Treatment of dementia. In: *Clinical Geriatric Psychopharmacology: Third Edition.* Edited by C. Salzman. Williams & Wilkins, Baltimore, Maryland (in press).
3. Becker, R.E. and Giacobini, E. Mechanisms of cholinesterase inhibition in senile dementia of the Alzheimer type: clinical, pharmacological, and therapeutic aspects. *Drug Dev Res* **12**, 163–195, 1988.
4. Cacabelos, R., Alvarez, X.A., Franco, M.A., *et al.* Effect of CDP-choline on cognition and immune function in Alzheimer's disease and multi infarct dementia. *Ann NY Acad Sci* **695**, 321–323, 1993.
5. Jorm, A.F. Effects of cholinergic enhancement therapies on memory function in Alzheimer's disease: a meta-analysis of the literature. *Aust New Zeal J Psychiatr* **20**, 237–240, 1986.

6. Davis, K.L., Thal, L.J., Gamzu, E., *et al.* Tacrine in patients with Alzheimer's disease: a double-blind, placebo-controlled multicenter study. *N Engl J Med* **327**, 1253–1259, 1992.

7. Enz, A. and Florshein, P. Cholinesterase inhibitors: an overview of their mechanisms of action. In: *Alzheimer Disease: From Molecular Biology to Therapy.* Edited by R. Becker, E. Giacobini. Birkhäuser Verlag AG, Boston, 1996, pp. 211–215.

8. Summers, W.K., Majovski, L.V., Marsh, G.M., *et al.* Oral tetrahydroaminoacridine in long-term treatment of senile dementia, Alzheimer type. *N Engl J Med* **315**, 1241–1245, 1986.

9. Schneider, L.S. Clinical pharmacology of aminoacridines in Alzheimer's disease. *Neurology* **43** (suppl. 4), S64–S79, 1993.

10. Schneider, L.S., and Forette, F. Alzheimer's disease symptomatic drugs: tacrine. In: *Clinical Diagnosis and Management of Alzheimer's Disease.* Edited by S. Gauthier. Martin Dunitz, London, 1996, pp. 221–237.

11. Eagger, S.A., Levy, R. and Sahakian, B.J. Tacrine in Alzheimer's disease. *Lancet* **337**, 989–992, 1991.

12. Farlow, M., Gracon, S.I., Hershey, L.A., *et al.* A 12-week, double-blind, placebo-controlled, parallel-group study of tacrine in patients with probable Alzheimer's disease. *JAMA* **268**, 2523–2529, 1992.

13. Wilcock, G.K., Surmon, D.J., Scott, M., *et al.* An evaluation of the efficacy and safety of tetrahydroaminoacridine (THA) without lecithin in the treatment of Alzheimer's disease. *Age Ageing* **22**, 316–324, 1993.

14. Knapp, M.J., Knopman, D.S., Solomon, P.R., *et al.* Controlled trials of high-dose tacrine in patients with Alzheimer's disease. *JAMA* **271**, 985–991, 1994.

15. Maltby, N., Broe, G.A., Creasey, H., *et al.* Efficacy of tacrine and lecithin in mild to moderate Alzheimer's disease: double blind trial. *Br Med J* **308**, 879–883, 1994.

16. Wood, P.C. and Castleden M. A double-blind, placebo controlled, multicenter study of tacrine for Alzheimer's disease. *Int J Geriatr Psychiatry* **9**, 649–654, 1994.

17. Antuono, P.G. Efficacy and safety of velnacrine for the treatment of Alzheimer's disease. A double-blind, placebo-controlled study. Mentane Study Group. *Arch Intern Med* **155**, 1766–1772, 1995.

18. Rogers, S.L. and Friedhoff, L. The efficacy and safety of donepezil in patients with Alzheimer's disease: results of a US multicentre, randomized, double-blind, placebo-controlled trial. *Dementia* **7**, 293–303, 1996.

19. Anand, R. and Gharabawi, G. Efficacy and safety results of the early phase studies with Exelon™ (ENA-713) in Alzheimer's disease: an overview. *J Drug Devel Clin Pract* **8**, 1–14, 1996.

20. Becker, R.E., Colliver, J.A., Markwell, S.J., *et al.* Double-blind, placebo-controlled study of metrifonate, an acetylcholinesterase inhibitor, for Alzheimer disease. *Alzheimer Dis Assoc Disorders* **10**, 124–131, 1996.

21. Morris, J., Cyrus, P., Orazem, J., Mas, J., Bieber, F. and Gulanski, B. Metrifonate: potential therapy for Alzheimer's disease. Poster Session at the American Academy of Neurology Annual Meeting, March 1997.

22. Canal, N., Imbimbo, B.P. and Lucchelli, P.E., for the Eptasigmine Study Group. A 25-week, double-blind, randomized, placebo-controlled, trial of eptastigmine in patients with diagnosis of probable Alzheimer's disease. *Eur J Neurol* **3** (suppl. 5), 238, 1996.

23. Fisher, A., Haring, R., Ginzburg, I., *et al.* Novel m1 muscarinic agonists: from symptomatic treatment to delaying the progression of Alzheimer's disease (AD). *Neurobiol Aging* **17** (4S), S48, 1996.

24. Thal, L.J., Masur, D.M., Sharpless, N.S., *et al*. Acute and chronic effects of oral physostigmine and lecithin in Alzheimer's disease. *Prog Neuropsychopharmacol Biol Psychiatry* **10**, 617–636, 1986.

25. Stern, Y., Sano, M. and Mayeux R. Long-term administration of oral physostigmine in Alzheimer's disease. *Neurology* **38**, 1837–1841, 1988.

26. Harrell, L.E., Callaway, R., Morere, D., and Falgout, J. The effect of long-term physostigmine administration in Alzheimer's disease. *Neurology* **40**, 1350–1354, 1990.

27. Beller, S.A., Overall, J.E., Rhoades, H.M., and Swann, A.C. Long-term outpatient treatment of senile dementia with oral physostigmine. *J Clin Psychiatry* **49**, 400–404, 1988.

28. Nordberg, A. Effect of long-term treatment with tacrine (THA) in Alzheimer's disease as visualized by PET. *Acta Neurol Scand* **149**, 62–65, 1993.

29. Wilcock, G.K., Scott, M. and Pearsall, T. Long-term use of tacrine. *Lancet* **343**, 294, 1994.

30. Knopman, D., Schneider, L., Davis, K., *et al*. Long-term tacrine treatment: effects on nursing home placement and mortality. *Neurology* **47**, 166–177, 1996.

31. Schneider, L.S. and Farlow, M.R. Predicting response to cholinesterase inhibitors in Alzheimer's disease: possible approaches. *CNS Drugs* **41**, 114–124, 1995.

32. Eagger, S., Morant, N., Levy, R. and Sahakian, B. Tacrine in Alzheimer's disease. Time course of changes in cognitive function and practice effects. *Br J Psychiatry* **160**, 36–40, 1992.

33. Schneider, L.S., Farlow, M.R., Henderson, V.W. and Pogoda, J.M. Effects of estrogen replacement therapy on response to tacrine in patients with Alzheimer's disease. *Neurology* **46**, 1580–1584, 1996.

34. Nordberg, A., Lilja, A., Lundqvist, H., *et al*. Tacrine restores cholinergic nicotinic receptors and glucose metabolism in Alzheimer patients as visualized by positron emission tomography. *Neurobiol Aging* **13**, 747–758, 1992.

35. Perryman, K.M. and Fitten, L.J. Delayed matching-to-sample performance during a double-blind trial of tacrine (THA) and lecithin in patients with Alzheimer's disease. *Life Sci* **53**, 479–486, 1993.

36. Farlow, M.R., Brashear, A., Hui, S., *et al*. for the Tacrine Study Group. The effects of tacrine in patients with mild versus moderate stage Alzheimer's disease. *Neurobiol Aging* **15** (suppl.), S81, 1995.

37. Raskind, M.A., Sadowsky, C.H., Sigmund, W.R., *et al*. Effect of tacrine on language, praxis and noncognitive behavioral problems in Alzheimer's disease. *Arch Neurol* (in press).

38. Olin, J.T. and Schneider, L.S. Assessing response to tacrine using the factor analytic structure of the Alzheimer's Disease Assessment Scale (ADAS)-cognitive subscale. *Int J Geriatr Psychiatry* **10**, 753–756, 1995.

39. Sahakian, B.J. and Coull, J.T. Tetrahydroaminoacridine (THA) in Alzheimer's disease: an assessment of attentional and mnemonic function using CANTAB. *Acta Neurol Scand* **149**, 29–35, 1993.

40. McKeith, I.G., Galasko, D., Kosaka, K., *et al*. Consensus guidelines for the clinical and pathologic diagnosis of dementia with Lewy bodies (DLB): report of the consortium on DLB international workshop. *Neurology* **47**, 1113–1124, 1996.

41. Levy, R., Eagger, S., Griffiths, M., *et al*. Lewy bodies and response to tacrine in Alzheimer's disease. *Lancet* **343**, 176, 1994.

42. Poirier, J., Dellsle, M.C. and Quirion, R. Apolipoprotein E4, cholinergic integrity, synaptic plasticity and Alzheimer's disease. In: *Apolipoprotein E and*

AD. Edited by A. Roses, K. Weisgraber, Y. Christian Springer-Verlag, New York, 1995, pp. 20–28.

43. Anand, R. and Enz, A. Clinical confirmation of preclinical attributes of ENA 713. Fifth International Conference on Alzheimer's Disease and Related Disorders. Osaka, Japan. July 24–29, 1996. *Neurobiol Aging* **17** (S4), S349, 1996.
44. Tariot, P.N., Schneider, L.S., Patel, S.V. and Goldstein B. Alzheimer's disease and (–)-deprenyl: rationale and findings. In: *Inhibitors of Monoamine Oxidase B Pharmacology and Clinical Use In Neurodegenerative Disorders*. Edited by I. Szelenyi. Birkhäuser Verlag AG, Basel, Switzerland, 1993, pp. 301–317.
45. Tariot, P.N. and Blazina, L. The psychopathology of dementia. In: *Handbook of Dementing Illnesses*. Edited by J.C. Morris. Marcell Dekker, New York, 1993, pp. 461–475.
46. Nyth, A.L. and Gottfries, C. The clinical efficacy of citalopram in treatment of emotional disturbances in dementia disorders: A Nordic Multicentre Study. *Br J Psychiatry* **157**, 894–901, 1990.
47. Cotman, C., Monaghan, D. and Ganong, A. Excitatory amino acid neurotransmission: NMDA receptors and Hebb-type synaptic plasticity. *Ann Rev Neurosci* **11**, 61–80, 1988.
48. Tatton, W.G. 'Trophic-like' reduction of nerve cell death by deprenyl without monoamine oxidase inhibition. *Neurol Forum* **4**, 3–10, 1993.
49. Cohen, G. and Spina, M.B. Deprenyl suppresses the oxidant stress associated with increased dopamine turnover. *Ann Neurol* **26**, 689–690, 1989.
50. Milgram, N.W., Racine, R.J., Nellis, P., *et al.* Maintenance on L-deprenyl prolongs life in aged male rats. *Life Sci* **47**, 415–420, 1990.
51. Sano, M., Ernesto, C., Klauber, M.R., *et al.* A two-year, double-blind randomized multicenter trial of selegiline and α-tocopherol in the treatment of Alzheimer's disease. *N Engl J Med* **336**, 1216–1222, 1997.
52. Gutzmann, H., Erzigkeit, H. and Hadler, D. Long-term treatment of Alzheimer's disease with idebenone. *Neurobiol Aging* **17** (4S), S141, 1996.
53. McGeer, P.L., McGeer, E., Rogers, J. and Sibley, J. Antiinflammatory drugs and Alzheimer's disease. *Lancet* **335**, 1037, 1987.
54. Breitner, J.C.S., Gau, B.A., Welsh, K.A., *et al.* Inverse association of anti-inflammatory treatments and Alzheimer's disease: initial results of a co-twin study. *Neurology* **44**, 227–232, 1994.
55. Rogers, J., Kirby, L.C., Hempelman, S.R., *et al.* Clinical trial of indomethacin in Alzheimer's disease. *Neurology* **43**, 1609–1611, 1993.
56. Aisen, P.S. and Davis, K.L. Inflammatory mechanisms in Alzheimer's disease: implications for therapy. *Am J Psychiatry* **151**, 1105–1113, 1994.
57. Tollefson, G.D. Short-term effects of the calcium channel blocker nimodipine (Bay-e9736) in the management of primary degenerative dementia. *Biol Psychiatry* **27**, 1133–1142, 1990.
58. Kanowski, S., Fischof, P., Hiersemenzel, R., *et al.* Wirksamkeitsnachweis von nootropika am beispiel von Nimodipin -ein beitrag zur entwicklung geeigneter klinischer prufmodelle. *Zeitscrift fur Gerontopsychologie und -psychiatrie* **1**, 35–44, 1988.
59. Hefti, F. and Schneider, L.S. Rationale for the planned clinical trials with nerve growth factor in Alzheimer's disease. *Psychiatric Devel* **4**, 297–315, 1989.
60. Olson, L. NGF and the treatment of Alzheimer's disease. *Exp Neurol* **124**, 5–15, 1993.
61. Schneider, L.S. and Finch, C. Can estrogen prevent neurodegeneration? *Drugs Aging* **11**(2), 87–95, 1997.

62. Parkinson, F.E., Rudolphi, K.A. and Fredholm, B.B. Propentofylline: a nucleo-side transport inhibitor with neuroprotective effects in cerebral ischemia. *Gen Pharmacol* **25**, 1053–1058, 1994.
63. Rother, M., Kittner, B., Rudolphi, K., Rossner, M. and Labs, K.H. HWA 285 (propentofylline) – a new compound for the treatment of both vascular dementia and dementia of the Alzheimer type. *Ann New York Acad Sci* **777**, 404–409, 1996.
64. Schneider, L.S. and Olin, J.T. Overview of clinical trials of Hydergine® in dementia. *Arch Neurol* **51**, 787–798, 1994.
65. Battaglia, A., Bruni, G., Ardia, A., *et al.* Nicergoline in mild to moderate dementia a multicenter, double-blind, placebo-controlled study. *J Am Geriatr Soc* **37**, 295–302, 1989.
66. Mondadori, C. Nootropics: preclinical results in the light of clinical effects; comparison with tacrine. *Crit Rev Neurobiol* **10**, 357–370, 1996.

7

Measuring memory

M.S. John Pathy

INTRODUCTION

The last 40 years has seen a progressive acceptance that dementia at any age is likely to have definable causes. This has encouraged renewed scientific interest in disorders associated with cognitive impairment. Clinical trials of an array of pharmaceutical compounds have underlined the need for study protocols to use standardised cognitive assessment instruments. The introduction of the cholinesterase inhibitor tetrahydroaminoacridine (tacrine) had a dramatic impact on public awareness of Alzheimer's disease in the USA: this heightened public awareness that the disorder is a relatively recent phenomenon in Europe.

Apart from serological (HIV, human immunodeficiency virus) tests for AIDS, now the commonest cause of dementia in young adults, there are no specific tests for most other causes of dementia. Memory impairment for recent events is the commonest and usually the earliest presenting feature of the dementia syndrome in the older population. This pivotal but non-specific marker may be determined by a multiplicity of factors including normal ageing. Elderly subjects' assessment of their memory is influenced by the types of questions posed or by their perception of memory changes. Memory self-assessment is often poor whereas relatives' opinion of memory impairment correlates closely with objective measures of memory. Informants' perceptions of cognitive deficits are often predictive of subsequent developments of probable Alzheimer's disease [1].

Psychopharmacology of Cognitive and Psychiatric Disorders in the Elderly. Edited by David Wheatley and David Smith. Published in 1998 by Chapman and Hall, London. ISBN 0 412 82470 1

MEMORY CLASSIFICATION

Memory tasks and processing are complex and multifactorial and the terminology and concepts used to describe these diverse aspects are confusing and subject to change.

The most frequently used model of memory function (embracing the initiating stimulus, consolidation, retention and retrieval) is based on an early concept of interrelated stores which has been subsequently modified to accommodate evidence of different types of memory processing. Information from sensory receptors, e.g. auditory, visual and tactile, triggers **sensory memory** processing; once information is perceived it is transferred to primary memory. It is more likely that sensory memory is a dynamic rather than a passive holding function and that it continues to operate for as long as the sensory stimulus requires ongoing analysis [2]. Memory storage is considered to be mediated by an encoding phenomenon. **Primary** memory (short term, immediate) functions as a limited capacity, brief holding stage where memory signals must be transferred to secondary (long-term) memory or reinforced by rehearsal if they are to be retained. In every day clinical practice short-term memory is often considered to represent memory for recent events measured over minutes or days; the term is so imprecise that it should be discarded. **Secondary** memory is conceived as a storage facility for consolidated memory of unlimited capacity and with a retention duration measured in hours to years. It has been postulated that remote memory may be held in some form of tertiary memory store that is more resistant to memory decay. The concept of working memory [3] has been put forward as a functional link between primary memory and ongoing memory processing.

A number of memory systems have been described and include:

- **semantic memory** (general knowledge) and **episodic memory** – recall of specific events [4]
- **procedural memory** – subconscious memory acquisition which may underpin several current functional skills [5]
- **perceptual representational memory** – subconscious acquisition of memory fragments which non-specifically augment memory tasks [6].

Lexical memory is regarded as a store for words or for their sound characteristics (phonemes) or written (graphemes) structure. The meaning of words depends on visual, auditory, tactile, gustatory, olfactory or perceptual information held in semantic memory. Memory organisation utilises **explicit memory** – conscious recognition of previously learned information/tasks and **implicit memory** – use of subconsciously learned information. Metamemory (knowledge of one's own memory capability) does not appear to be significantly affected by age [7]. Focal brain lesions, e.g. temporal lobe involvement, may impair some aspects of metamemory.

Processing resources (and their many variants including reduced inhibitory capacity, e.g. for attentional competition) are conceived as capacity functions which impact on memory and may be enhanced or impaired by environmental factors. A recent study on retrieval efficiency [8] supports the resource reduction hypothesis.

AGEING AND COGNITIVE FUNCTION

Complaints of memory impairment are common in otherwise independently living older people. Most published reports of the influence of ageing on memory have been cross-sectional in design and few have included subjects of advanced age. The distinction between age-related (differences between defined chronological groups) and ageing-related (due to an ageing process) memories is often unclear. Primary memory appears to remain intact in normal ageing [9]. The reported effect of age on working memory has been somewhat contradictory but there is now general agreement that elderly individuals function as well as young adults in simple tasks such as digit span but less well with complex tasks [10], probably due to impairment of processing speed [11]. Increased distractability may affect the ageing memory [12]. Impairment of name recall (semantic memory) is a common complaint in old age, yet many tests of semantic memory show little or no age-related change. Free recall tests, e.g. generating a list of flowers or animal names in a given time or recalling a word list, does appear to decline with age but predominantly after age 70 years [13]. Ageing differences in secondary memory have been postulated as being due to a reduction in processing resources [14,15] or reduced inhibitory functioning [12], allowing intrusions and thus distractions in memory processing. Remote memory is said to show little decline with age but because of the multiplicity of factors that influence past memories it is extremely difficult to test. Studies variably show no decline [16], intermittent stages of decline [17] or a comparative decline between young and old adults when tested on a series of present to past memories [18].

The storage model of memory is a highly stylised framework which together with associated encoding and retrieval phenomena serves to focus on some of the main aspects of memory function. Memory is not an isolated function, however, but it is influenced by other cognitive domains, e.g. intelligence, reasoning, perception, language and spatial abilities. Intelligence and memory are not always parallel phenomena even in old age [19]. Tests of reasoning and spatial ability show some decline with age [20]. Language is a highly complex cognitive function and forms the main channel for communicating human thoughts. Impaired naming ability, which may be due to retrieval problems [21,22] or a slowing of lexical accessing [23], is the commonest age-related language change. An apparent decline of syntactic performance with age is probably due to an impaired ability of the working memory to simultaneously hold and process complex sentences [24].

ASSESSMENT OF COGNITIVE FUNCTION

The debate continues as to whether dementia is one extreme of a distribution on normal ageing [25] or a distinct disease [26]. What is clear is that cognitive function instruments, particularly screening tests, show an overlap between early dementia and normal ageing.

The determination of cognitive competence and the evaluation of evidence of dementia is dependent on a balanced amalgam of clinical assessment and neuropsychological tests. Indeed, some test instruments, e.g. CAMDEX (Cambridge Mental Disorders of the Elderly Examination) [27], include a structured interview with both the patient and an informant together with a battery of mini mental function tests. Clinical examination supported by a detailed and probing history from both patient and informant will usually clarify symptoms of cognitive impairment. Subtle changes of lifestyle, an account of unexpected redundancy or premature retirement, isolated episodes of orientation difficulties in a holiday hotel, perhaps a few years earlier, or minor changes in driving patterns, such as hesitancy at roundabouts, may be important but easily overlooked markers of early cognitive dysfunction. A counsel of perfection is unrealistic in many scenarios, however, as informants may be unavailable and time is often limited. Even with detailed assessment the significance of mild memory loss may be unascertainable on a single visit: change over time may provide the only certain evidence of cognitive decline.

MENTAL TEST SCREENING INSTRUMENTS

The purposes for which a neuropsychological test or battery of tests are required should determine the relevant instrument. In everyday practice simple screening tests which can be administered in less than 10 minutes are often used to support the presence or absence of cognitive impairment. Other tests may have different or additional aims, e.g. diagnostic, staging or grading the severity of established dementia. Screening tests are not intended to be diagnostic instruments: they have an important role in alerting the busy clinician or in supporting an historical evaluation of cognitive complaints as well as providing a recorded measure of mental status.

The use of an overall test score can blur specific deficits. Screening tests measure particular types of memory and cannot provide a global assessment of memory function. Premorbid intelligence and educational background may enable a normal score to be achieved despite early dementia (ceiling effect), and where dementia is severe it may not be possible to demonstrate further deterioration (floor effect). Indeed the case control study method used in developing many screening tests excludes the earliest features of cognitive change. The tests either ignore temporal components or, if a time restriction is included, e.g. Kendrick Digit Copying Task [28], the results may be influenced by changes in manual dexterity due to physical disorders rather than cognitive impairment. Individual components of screening tests that cover several cognitive domains are often insufficiently detailed to clarify a complaint of mild memory impairment.

The syndrome of dementia as based on DSM IV (Diagnostic and Statistical Manual of the American Psychiatric Association 4th edition) [29] and the ICD 10 (International Classification of Disease, 10th revision) [30] criteria cannot be diagnosed by testing a single cognitive domain. A high degree of discrimination between normal elderly subjects and demented individuals was achieved from a community study by summing the scores of object recall and face-associated name recall tests [31]. The early neuronal changes that occur in the medio-temporal lobe and particularly the hippocampal region of the brain in Alzheimer's disease are associated with impaired tests of explicit memory. As progressive change occurs in the neocortex evidence of more global cognitive deficits becomes apparent.

Confounding factors

Environmental and psychological circumstances may have a substantial impact on cognitive function [32,33]. The influence of the visual environment on visual performance tasks [34] is often substantial and frequently disregarded. Patients with Alzheimer's disease have a high prevalence of hearing loss which they report less often than healthy control subjects [35], and yet hearing ability is rarely tested prior to cognitive assessment procedures. Screening tests are often performed under a variety of circumstances where lighting is variable, noise may be prominent and distraction is often unavoidable. Many therapeutic agents may impair memory, e.g. benzodiazepines, anti-Parkinsonian, hypotensive and anti-muscarinic agents are common offenders.

Mini Mental State Examination (MMSE)

This internationally accepted cognitive screening instrument of 30 items (MMSE [36]) covers orientation in person, place and time, short-term recall, comprehension, language, attention and construction. The test is primarily used to obtain an overall score as an indicator of the presence and severity of dementia. Despite the reported poor discriminatory ability of the three-word recall task [37], performance on individual components often provides valuable information that is too often disregarded. The original cut-off score of 20 has been revised to 23 to improve sensitivity while attempting to maintain reasonable specificity. Age [38] and education and social class [39] significantly influence the cut-off point used to denote cognitive impairment.

The full version of the Serial Sevens Test required the serial subtraction of seven from 100 in 14 consecutive steps. The shortened version of five serial subtractions of seven was incorporated into the original MMSE, whilst substitution of the word WORLD to be spelt backwards was to be exceptional. Commonly the two tasks have been considered comparable and optional but correlation is weak [40] and Ganguli and her colleagues [41] found that 25% of subjects scored 5 points lower with Serial Seven tasks than with the WORLD backward version. These authors also point to the lack of standard guidelines for scoring WORLD backwards.

Attempts to separate the effects of normal ageing from early dementia have led to the development of slightly more complex yet reasonably brief screening tests using one of three approaches: respondent administered tests, a mixture of administered and informant derived scales or informant based tests.

Blessed Dementia Scale (BDS)

This scale [42] is in two parts:

1. An informant derived and rated information of daily living activities, personal habits (eating, dressing and sphincter control) and changes in personality, interests and drive.
2. An administered Information-Memory-Concentration Test. This instrument has been widely used in dementia research and appears sensitive to changes in dementia severity [43] but both the functional rating scale [44] and the Information-Memory-Concentration Test appear to have ceiling effects [44] and probably floor effects [45].

Abbreviated Mental Test (AMT)

This test [46] is widely used in the UK for the rapid assessment of cognitive status. The 10 items, derived from the 38-item Roth-Hopkins Test, include orientation in time, place and person, secondary and remote memory, understanding and attention. An original cut-off score of 7 was considered as indicative of cognitive impairment. In a comparative study of the CAMCOG (Cognitive Section of CAMDEX), MMSE, cognitive items of CAPE (Clifton Assessment Procedure for the Elderly) [47] and Blessed Dementia Scale, an AMT score of 8/8.5 had a sensitivity of 93.5% and a specificity of 87% in separating normals from the cognitively impaired [48]. The AMT is a screening instrument to indicate moderate dementia but it is not sufficiently sensitive to identify mild cognitive impairment. As the test items can be committed to memory it is used in a variety of settings. The omission of individual components seriously impairs the validity of the cut-off point [49].

Short Portable Mental Status Questionnaire

The 10-point questionnaire [50] was established as a brief screening instrument suitable for multi-situational use, e.g. community, outpatient clinics or institutional settings. The test items focus on orientation, short-term and remote memory, current events, calculation and a question relevant to self-care. The test was designed to be suitable for elderly subjects and to identify global cognitive impairment: a score of more than five errors represents significant impairment.

Brief Cognitive Rating Scale (BCRS)

The BCRS [51] assesses five domains:
- concentration (Axis I),
- recent memory (Axis II),
- past memory (Axis III),
- orientation (Axis IV)
- function and self-care (Axis V).

Each domain has a 7-point rating scale and an overall score of 5 represents no cognitive abnormality and a score of 35 indicates severe dementia. The BCRS has the advantage that subjective impairment or early features of cognitive dysfunction can be identified and either serves as a marker for future follow-up and reassessment or calls for more detailed neuropsychological testing. The test requires some input from an informant. The test can normally be administered in 15 minutes. Test results may be within the normal range in individuals of above average intelligence who present with complaints of early memory impairment. The addition of delayed free recall tests should extend the sensitivity of the instrument.

Short Test of Mental Status (STMS)

The STMS [52] provides more information than the MMSE and contains items on orientation, attention, immediate recall, calculation, abstraction, construction, and information and recall with a total score of 38. A cut-off point of 29 has been shown to have a sensitivity of 86.4% in identifying dementia and a specificity of 88.4%. The test has a high correlation with the MMSE, the Blessed Information-Memory-Concentration Test, the Mattis Dementia Rating Scale [53] and the WAIS R [54].

Informant Questionnaire on Cognitive Decline in the Elderly (IQCODE)

This test [55] is based on a 26-item questionnaire which is administered to an informant who is asked to quantify the levels of change of memory and intelligence for a variety of situations over the previous 10 years [56]. The test compares favourably with the MMSE and is not obviously influenced by educational background, which is a substantial weakness of many screening instruments. The IQCODE cut-off point of 3.6 gives a reasonable degree of sensitivity without an undue number of false positives. The applicability of the test as a screening tool is limited by the availability of an informant with 10 years' knowledge of the subject.

TESTS OF MEMORY FUNCTION

Complaints of altered memory function are a feature of a variety of cognitive and non-cognitive conditions. The memory sections of many screening tests are too limited to provide an adequate assessment of memory function. Selection of a memory instrument will be suggested by (1) clinical information supplemented by a brief general cognitive screening test and (2) answers to relevant questions: Is memory impaired? If memory function is impaired, are other cognitive functions affected? How severe is memory impairment?

Wechsler Memory Scale – Revised (1987)

This scale [57] is the standard instrument for assessing a wide spectrum of memory functions but requires to be administered by trained psychologists. It has been designed to be compatible with the WAIS-R (Wechsler Adult Intelligence Scale – Revised). In essence it consists of introductory questions on personal and current information and on orientation to provide an assessment of the respondent's potential to undertake the complete test. The 12 individual subtests cover five major areas of memory function: memory control (attention and concentration), i.e. counting from 20 to 1; reciting the alphabet and a serial three counting task from 1 to 40 to time; verbal memory: (1) logical memory tested by immediate recall of two stories and (2) associate learning using paired word tests with practice repeats to assess learning ability; visual memory tested by (1) recognition of a previously studied geometrical shape from an array of several similar shapes, (2) a paired line drawings-colour recall with subsequent presentation of line drawings only. Delayed memory recall (30 minutes) is derived from recall of the verbal and visual memory procedures.

The WMS-R has well-established norms and provides an assessment of immediate and delayed recall of both verbal and non-verbal stimuli. The test requires active respondent participation and vigilance on the part of the examiner. The battery type memory instruments test a range of memory functions but the summing of raw scores to form a derived memory index has the inherent risk of blurring the influence of individual components. Scrutiny of each function tested, e.g. primary memory (a highly attention-dependent function), permits appropriate interpretation of the derived memory index. A number of briefer memory tests have been introduced which have a wider application and can often be used by trained non-psychologists.

Word Recall Test (WRT) from the CERAD

This test [58] has been shown to have high sensitivity and specificity in separating early Alzheimer's disease from normal controls but poor discriminatory ability in separating mild from moderate Alzheimer's disease [59]. The WRT is essentially a 10-word list memory test of immediate free recall and delayed recall after five to eight minutes. The combination of a delayed word recognition test (test words and distracter words) and the WRT appears to afford greater accuracy in discriminating between moderate and severe Alzheimer's disease [59].

Three Shapes Three Words Mental State Test

This test [60] requires the immediate and delayed recall (15 minutes) of three shapes and three words. The test has the advantage of assessing visual perceptual processing; educational background and intelligence status appear to have minimal impact on performance.

Camden Memory Test

This test [61] provides five standardised and validated individual memory tests to cover several aspects of memory function:

- Pictorial recognition memory test for detecting functional memory deficits. This is useful in identifying false claims of memory impairment.
- Topographical recognition memory test is designed to test topographical memory particularly in unilateral brain lesions.
- Paired associate learning test is less susceptible to floor/ceiling effects than the Wechsler Paired Associate Test.
- Short recognition memory test for words.
- Short recognition test for faces.
  Both (4) and (5) are sensitive to stages of cognitive decline.

As indicated earlier, screening tests are not intended to be diagnostic instruments but are designed to signal cognitive impairment. Test scores for normal elderly subjects and mildly demented individuals often overlap. Most brief screening tests are predominantly verbal in structure which may introduce educational bias. Discriminatory power and diagnostic supplementation may be achieved by more detailed neuropsychological and interview assessment.

Dementia Rating Scale (DRS)

Although this instrument [53] has been used as a more sophisticated screening test, it was designed to be sensitive to longitudinal changes in cognitive decline in an elderly population. The validity of the total DRS score in staging the progress of dementia has been confirmed by Shay and her colleagues [62]. The absence of significant floor effect is a major advantage of this test when measuring decline in severe dementia. The DRS subscales essentially correspond to attention (8 items), initiation/perseveration (11 items), construction (6 items), conceptualisation (6 items) and memory (5 items). The DRS has a total score of 144 and a cut-off score of 123 represents the presence of cognitive impairment. The author suggests that it takes 10–15 minutes to administer the test in normal elderly individuals, and 30–45 minutes for demented patients.

Kendrick Battery – Revised

This battery [28] is based on a neuropsychological-behavioural concept and its original strategic aim was to distinguish drug-related pseudodementia from demented and non-demented elderly subjects. The revised version of the battery comprises the object learning test and the digit copying test. These two components were never intended to be used separately but the digit copying test component has been used to increase the discriminatory power of other brief screening tests. It is a timed instrument and tests sensorimotor function, which is probably dependent on CNS functional competency and speed. In essence, the respondent copies as many of the 100 numbers given as quickly as possible within two minutes. To overcome ceiling effects, the task is also measured in seconds for those who manage to copy all 100 figures in less than the target period. The raw scores are age scaled and unlike the digit substitution tests of the WAIS scale, which has a floor effect in more severe stages of dementia, the digit copying test often continues to provide a marker of deterioration.

Gottfries, Brane, Steen Scale (GBS)

This scale [63] was primarily constructed for measuring dementia syndromes in hospital or other institutional settings and can be performed by nurses, psychologists and physicians. The GBS provides a validated, comprehensive but manageable instrument with four main subscales covering:

- motor functions (activities of daily living including sphincter control)
- intellectual (orientation, recent memory, remote memory, wakefulness, concentration, competence with tempo, absent-mindedness, long-windedness, distractability)
- emotional functions (blunting, lability, motivation)
- symptoms common in dementia syndrome (confusion, irritability, anxiety, agony, reduced mood, restlessness).

The emotional impairment component probably requires training to a common protocol to establish a high correlation between physicians, psychologists and nurses.

CAMDEX (Cambridge Mental Disorders of the Elderly Examination)

This standardised instrument [27] was devised for the diagnosis of mental disorders in elderly subjects with particular emphasis on the early diagnosis of dementia and has been used in epidemiological studies. The design of the instrument seeks to provide a cohesive and integrated schedule for the diagnosis of both the presence and category of dementia as a measure of the severity and extent of cognitive impairment and to rate behaviour and everyday activities. The CAMDEX schedule has seven sections but the three main areas comprise a standard clinical interview with the patient and a structured interview with an informant and a mini battery of brief cognitive tests (CAMCOG). The CAMCOG tests orientation, language, memory, praxis, attention, abstract thinking, perception and calculation. A complete schedule (other than radiological tests) can be completed in approximately 80 minutes, of which about 20 minutes is spent on the informant interview.

The CAMCOG section has been shown to be a reliable procedure for dementia discrimination in an elderly population and, with a cut-off score of 69/70, has a sensitivity of 97% and a specificity of 91% for moderate/severe dementia [48]. Age, education, hearing and vision have a significant effect on this instrument.

Wechsler Adult Intelligence Scale Revised – incorporating British amendments to the text and administration section (WAIS-R UK).

This instrument [54] is widely used by psychologists on both sides of the Atlantic and measures intelligence against recorded norms (derived from North American subjects). All scores are scaled and adjusted for age up to 75 years. The WAIS-R yields an IQ score and, if used in association with a predictive test of premorbid intelligence, e.g. NART [64], provides an invaluable measure of intellectual decline. The 11 subscales cover a wide range of cognitive function and the test items in each subscale are progressively graded in terms of difficulty. Six of the tests are grouped into a verbal scale and five are performance tests. The tests are administered in a given order to allow comparability with established norms. The verbal tests include:

- information,
- comprehension,
- arithmetic,
- similarities,
- digit span,
- vocabulary and performance tests,
- digit symbol,
- picture completion,
- block design,
- picture arrangement,
- picture assembly.

Each of the 11 tests contains items of increasing order of difficulty. For example, information contains 29 questions. The instrument effectively identifies several areas of cognition and is sensitive to cognitive change over time.

Alzheimer's Disease Assessment Scale (ADAS)

This scale [65] was designed specifically for psychopharmacological research in Alzheimer's disease and was constructed around the cognitive and non-cognitive behavioural characteristics of this disorder. It does not follow that the ADAS is without application in assessing the progress of vascular dementia: it was not intended to be a diagnostic instrument. The scale appears to be a sensitive predictor of change in Alzheimer's disease [66]. The ADAS has two broad categories of cognitive and non-cognitive scales:

1. The cognitive component tests:
   (a) memory (ten word – three attempts – recall task, 12 word – three attempts – recognition task and a task instruction recognition item)
   (b) language (expressive, receptive, word-finding, object naming and a semi-structural interview to rate nine expressive and receptive language items)
   (c) tests of ideational and praxis and constructional ability.
2. The non-cognitive component consists of 23 items that evaluate mood state and assess behavioural disorders. The scale for the cognitive component is 0–70 and for the non-cognitive subscale is 0–25.

The ADAS test can be completed in 45 minutes but many elderly patients take considerably longer, especially on the constructional test, and they often dislike the three trials of the word recall and word recognition test. Test fatigue is a problem for some old people.

Clinical Dementia Rating (CDR)

Multi-centre trials are now the established method for evaluating the efficacy of new therapeutic agents in dementia research. A fundamental variable is the stage of the disorder. Assessment of dementia severity requires a defined protocol and a precise scoring method. The CDR [67,68] was developed as a staging instrument for longitudinal studies on patients with mild Alzheimer's disease. Six cognitive domains – memory, orientation, judgement and problem-solving, community affairs, home and hobbies, and personal care – are scored on a scale of 0, 0.5, 1, 2, 3. 0 is no loss, 0.5 questionable and 1–3 mild to severe impairment. The score for each category is derived from all available information – structured and unstructured interview with respondent and informant. Memory is a primary category and all other components are secondary. The rules for arriving at a final score have been published [67].

Cognitive impairment will influence the ability to function competently in some or many aspects of daily living. Instrumental activities of daily living are assessed in some of the global scales described above but there are occasions when it is appropriate to include an informant-based IADL Scale (Instrumental Activity of Daily Living) with one of the brief screening cognitive instruments. A number of scales are available, an appropriate one being the following.

Interview for Deterioration in Daily Functioning in Dementia (IDD) [69]

This explores 33 self-care activities and their performance initiative by a structured interview with a caregiver. The activities include personal functioning, e.g. washing, dressing and eating, and more involved activities, e.g. use of telephone, shopping and writing. The caregiver is asked to compare, on a three-point scale, the frequency of help provided compared with the help required prior to the onset of symptoms. The overall score ranges from 33 for no deterioration to 99 for gross deterioration.

DEPRESSION

Complaints of memory impairment occur with major depression but are particularly common in old people with milder depressive symptoms. Depressive features may also be prominent in the dementia syndrome.

Hamilton Depression Rating Scale (HDRS)

This rating scale [70] is the most widely used instrument for primary depressive illness. The HDRS was designed to provide a total score for 17 of its 21 items but all 21 items are used by some investigators. Some of the 17 items are rated on a 0–4 scale and others on a 0–2 scale. Rating consistency between observers is improved by using a structured interview guide [71]. Attempts have been made to improve the reliability of some items of this scale. The HDRS was designed to be administered by a skilled observer after a 30-minute interview.

Geriatric Depression Scale (GDS)

This provides a useful screening instrument [72] for self-administration or administration by untrained observers. The 30 questions which each have Yes/No answers were selected to be relevant to depression in elderly people. A 'Yes' response to 20 questions and a 'No' response to 10 questions indicate the presence of depression. A cut-off score of 11 on the GDS has an 84% sensitivity and 95% specificity, whilst a cut-off score of 14 has an 80% sensitivity but no false positives – 100% specificity. The GDS can be administered by untrained staff in a variety of settings and forms a useful screening test for depression in elderly individuals.

Hospital Anxiety and Depression Scale (HAD)

Emotional disorders in old people are a presenting complaint of memory disturbance. The HAD [73] was initially introduced as a brief validated self-assessment screening instrument for patients attending outpatient clinics but it has subsequently been validated for community use. The HAD scale contains seven items in each anxiety-depression subscale. The 14 items are graded 0–3 for severity, with 0 = no symptoms. A score range of 10/11 produces few false positives but a score range of 8/9 increases the sensitivity (i.e. low proportion of false negatives.)

INTELLECTUAL AND GLOBAL

National Adult Reading Test (NART) – Revised

Premorbid intelligence substantially influences the results of many cognitive function tests and brief screening instruments are particularly susceptible to intellectual ability. The NART (revised version) [64] is a validated and reliable measure of premorbid intelligence. Word reading ability shows substantial correlation with general intelligence. Accurately reading aloud English words that do not follow the rules of pronunciation requires previous knowledge of the words. Nelson [64] devised a list of 50 words that do not follow the normal rules of pronunciation and they are administered in order of increasing difficulty. The number of errors of pronunciation are recorded and a predicted full scale IQ, a predicted verbal IQ and a predicted performance IQ can be calculated. Discrepancy between the WAIS-R full scale IQ and the NART predicted full scale IQ is a measure of intellectual decline. The test appears to be a valid instrument for use in adults of all ages up to the middle of the ninth decade.

Objective mental status instruments are fundamental for evaluating psychopharmacological agents, but global clinical assessment of change embraces nuances of behaviour or function that may be impractical to incorporate into rating scales. The FDA (Food and Drug Administration – US 1990) guidelines for anti-dementia drug evaluation recommend inclusion of clinical global assessment of change over time [74].

Clinician Interview Based Impression (CIBI)

The CIBI has been designed as an instrument to assess global change. The CIBI rates change from baseline on a (1) very much improved to (7) very much worse scale and has the intermediate score of (4) to indicate no change. The CIBI has been shown to be a useful, albeit not very sensitive, instrument for evaluating cognitive change [74]. A number of changes, particularly inclusion of descriptors, have been proposed to clarify the basis on which the clinical process is determined [74].

Memory tests have strengths and weaknesses

The tests described are structured, validated and standardised with established norms. The test procedures allow comparison between different observers and institutions and they provide a reliable temporal record. Minor modifications have been necessary for some tests to take account of cultural or national differences, e.g. WAIS-R UK edition. Tests may be influenced by observer–respondent interactions and computerised memory tests have been introduced to overcome examiner variables [75]. Neuropsychological tests, however, cannot adequately account for the nuances imposed by culture, family, social interactions and environment. Psychopharmacological research has attempted to address the complexities of cognitive, functional and social factors in elderly individuals with memory impairment by using a range of tests that may extend over an hour and a half. The very real element of patient fatigue is too often overlooked.

REFERENCES

1. Tierney M.C., Szalai J.P., Snow W.G. Fisher R.H. The Prediction of Alzheimer's Disease. The Role of Patient and Informant Perception of Cognitive Deficits. *Archives of Neurology* 1966, **53**, 423–427.
2. D-Lollo B., Armett J.L., Cruk R.V. Age-Related Changes in the Rate of Visual Information Processing. *Journal of Experimental Psychology*: *Human Perception and Performance* 1982, **8**, 225–237.
3. Baddeley A. Working Memory. *Science* 1992, **255**, 556–559.
4. Tulving E. Episodic and Semantic Memory. In: E. Tulving and W. Donaldson (eds). *Organisation of Memory*, 1972, pp. 382–404. Academic Press, New York.
5. Tulving E., Schacter D.L. Priming and Human Memory Systems. *Science* 1990, **247**, 301–306.
6. Tulving E., Schacter D.L., Stark A.J. Priming Effects of Word-Fragment Completion are Independent of Recognition Memory. *Journal of Experimental Psychology*: *Learning, Memory, and Cognition* 1982, **8**, 336–342.
7. Hultsch D.F., Hertzog C., Dixon R.A. Age Differences in Metamemory: Resolving the Inconsistencies. *Canadian Journal of Psychology* 1987, **41**, 193–208.
8. Fastenau P.S., Denburg N.L., Abeles N. Age Differences in Retrieval: Further Support for the Resource-Reduction Hypothesis. *Psychology and Aging* 1996, **11**, 140–146.
9. Craik F.I.M., Jennings J.M. Human Memory. In: F.I.M. Craik and T.A. Salthouse (eds). *A Handbook of Aging and Cognition*, 1992. LEA, New Jersey.
10. Craik F.I.M., Morris R.G., Glick M.L. Adult Age Differences in Working Memory. In: G Vallar and T Shallice (eds). *Neuropscyhological Impairments of Short Term Memory*, 1990, pp. 247–267. Cambridge University Press, Cambridge.
11. Salthouse T.A., Babcock R.L. Decomposing Adult Age Differences in Working Memory. *Developmental Psychology* 1991, **27**, 763–776.
12. Hasher L., Zacks R.T. Working Memory, Comprehension, and Aging: A Review and a New View. In: G.H. Bower (ed). *The Psychology of Learning and Motivation*, 1988, Vol. 22. pp. 193–225. Academic Press, New York.
13. Albert M.S. Age-Related Changes in Cognitive Function. In: F.A. Huppert, C. Brayne and D.W. O'Connor (eds). *Dementia and Normal Aging*, 1994, pp. 291–329. Cambridge University Press, Cambridge.
14. Craik F.I.M., Byrd M. Ageing and Cognitive Deficits: The Role of Attentional Resources. In: F.I.M. Craik and S. Trehub (eds). *Aging and Cognitive Processes*, 1982, pp. 191–211. Plenum Press, New York.
15. Salthouse T.A. Resource-Reduction Interpretations of Cognitive Aging. *Developmental Review* 1988, 238–272.
16. Howes J.L., Katz A.N. Assessing Remote Memory with an Improved/Public Events Questionnaire. *Psychology and Aging* 1988, **3**, 142–150.
17. Bahrick H.P. Maintainance of Knowledge: Questions About Memory We Forgot To Ask. *Journal of Experimental Psychology*: *General* 1979, **108**, 296–308.
18. Rubin D.C., Wetzler S.E., Neebes R.D. Autobiographic Memory Across the Lifespan. In: D.C. Rubin (ed). *Autobiographical Memory*, 1986. Cambridge University Press, Cambridge.
19. Cockburn J., Smith P.T. The Relative Influence of Intelligence and Age on Everyday Memory. *Journal of Gerontology*: *Psychological Sciences* 1991, **46**, 31–36.
20. Salthouse T.A. Reasoning and Spatial Abilities. In: F.I.M. Craik and T.A. Salthouse (eds). *Handbook of Aging and Cognition*, 1992, pp. 167–211. LEA, New Jersey.

21. Burke D.M., Mackay D.G., Worthley J.A., Wade E. On the Tip of the Tongue: What Causes Word-finding Failures in Young and Older Adults? *Journal of Memory and Language* 1991, **30**, 542–579.
22. Light L.L. The Organisation of Memory in Old Age. In: F.I.M. Craik and T.A. Salthouse (eds). *Handbook of Aging and Cognition*, 1992, pp.111–165. LEA, New Jersey.
23. Balota D.A., Ducek J.M. Age-Related Differences in Lexical Access: Spreading Activation and Simple Pronunciation. *Psychology of Aging* 1988, **3**, 84–93.
24. Light L.L. Memory and Aging: Four Hypotheses in Search of Data. *Annual Review of Psychology* 1991, **42**, 333–376.
25. Huppert F.A., Brayne C. What is the Relationship Between Dementia and Normal Aging? In: F.A. Huppert, C. Brayne and D.W. O'Connor (eds). *Dementia and Normal Ageing*, 1994, pp. 3–11. Cambridge University Press, Cambridge.
26. Ritchie K., Kildea D. Is Senile Dementia "Age-Related or Ageing-Related?" Evidence from Meta-analysis of Dementia Prevalence in the Oldest Old. *Lancet* 1995, **346**, 931–934.
27. Roth M., Tym E., Mountjoy E.Q., *et al.* CAMDEX. A Standardised Instrument of the Diagnosis of Mental Disorder in the Elderly with Special Reference to Early Detection of Dementia. *British Journal of Psychiatry* 1986, **149**, 698–709.
28. Kendrick D.C., Gibson A.J., Moyes I.C.A. The Revised Kendrick Battery: Clinical Studies. *British Journal of Social and Clinical Psychology* 1979, **18**, 329–340.
29. *Diagnostic and Statistical Manual of Mental Disorders*, fourth edition, 1994. American Psychiatric Association, Washington DC.
30. *The ICD 10 Classification of Mental and Behavioural Disorders*, 1993. World Health Organization, Geneva.
31. Huppert F.A., Beardsall L. A Comparison of Clinical, Psychometric and Behavioural Memory Tests: Findings from a Community Study of the Early Detection of Dementia. *International Journal of Geriatric Psychiatry* 1991, **6**, 295–306.
32. Winocur G., Moscovitch M. Paired-Associate Learning in Institutionalised and Non-Institutionalised Old People. *Journal of Gerontology* 1984, **38**, 455–464.
33. Winocur G., Moscovitch M. A Comparison of Cognitive Function In Institutionalised and Community-Dwelling Old People of Normal Intelligence. *Canadian Journal of Psychology* 1990, **44**, 435–444.
34. Charness N., Bosman F.A. Human Factors and Design for Older Adults. In: J.E. Birren and K.W. Schaie (eds). *Handbook of the Psychology of Aging*, 1990, 3rd edition, pp. 446–463. Academic Press, San Diego.
35. Gold M., Lightfoot L.A., Hnatth-Chisholm T. Hearing Loss in Memory Disorders Clinic. A Specially Vulnerable Population. *Archives of Neurology* 1996, **53**, 922–928.
36. Folstein M.F., Folstein S.E., McHughe P.R. Mini Mental State Examination. A Practical Method for Grading the Cognitive State of patients for the Clinician. *Journal of Psychiatric Research* 1975, **12**, 189–198.
37. Huppert F.A. Memory Function in Dementia and Normal Aging – Dimension or Dichotomy? In: F.A. Huppert, C. Brayne and D.W. O'Connor (eds). *Dementia and Normal Aging*, 1994, pp. 291–330. Cambridge University Press, Cambridge.
38. Bleecker M.L., Bowla-Wilson K., Kawas C., Agnew J. Eight Specific Norms for the Mini Mental State Exam. *Neurology* 1988, **38**, 1565–1568.
39. O'Connor D.W., Pollitt P.A., Treasure T., *et al.* The Influence of Education, Social Class and Sex on Mini Mental State Scores. *Psychological Medicine* 1989, **19**, 771–776.

40. Holzer C.E., Tischler G.L., Leaf P.J., *et al*. An Epidemiological Assessment of Cognitive Impairment in a Community Population. In: J.R. Greenley (ed). *Research In Community and Mental Health*, 1984, p. 3. JAI Press, Greenwich.
41. Ganguli M., Ratcliff G., Huff J., *et al*. Serial Sevens versus WORLD Backwards: A Comparison of the Two Measures of Attention from the MMSE. *Journal of Geriatric Psychiatry and Neurology* 1990, **3**, 203–207.
42. Blessed G., Tomlinson B., Roth M. The Association Between Quantitative Measures of Dementia and of Senile Changes in the Cerebral Grey Matter of Elderly Subjects. *British Journal of Psychiatry* 1968, **114**, 797–811.
43. Uhlmann R.F., Larson E.B., Buchner D.M. Correlations of Mini Mental State and Modified Dementia Rating Scale to Measures of Transitional Health Status in Dementia. *Journal of Gerontology* 1987, **42**, 33–36.
44. Katzman R., Brown T., Thal L.J., *et al*. Comparison of Rate of Annual Change in Mental Status Score in Four Independent Studies of Patients with Alzheimer's Disease. *Annals of Neurology* 1988, **24**, 384–389.
45. Salmon D.P., Thal L.J., Butters N., Heindel W.C. Longitudinal Evaluation of Dementia of the Alzheimer's Type: A Comparison of Three Standardised Mental Status Examinations. *Neurology* 1990, **40**, 1225–1230.
46. Hodkinson H.M. Evaluation of a Mental Test Score for Assessment of Mental Impairment in the Elderly. *Age and Ageing* 1972, **1**, 233–238.
47. Pattie A.H., Gilleard C.J. The Clifton Assessment Schedule – Further Validation of a Psychogeriatric Assessment Schedule. *British Journal of Psychiatry* 1976, **129**, 68–72.
48. Blessed G., Black S.E., Butler T., Kay D.W. The Diagnosis of Dementia in the Elderly: A Comparison of CAMCOG (the cognitive section of CAMDEX), the AGECAT Programme, DSM III, The Mini Mental State Examination and Some Short Rating Scales. *British Journal of Psychiatry* 1991, **195**, 193–198.
49. Holmes J., Gilbody S. Differences in Use of Abbreviated Mental Test Scores by Geriatricians and Psychiatrists. *British Medical Journal* 1996, **313**, 465.
50. Pfeiffer E. A Short Portable Mental Status Questionnaire for the Assessment of Organic Brain Deficit in Elderly Patients. *Journal of the American Geriatrics Society* 1975, **23**, 433–441.
51. Reisberg B., Ferris F.H. Brief Cognitive Rating Scale (BCRS). *Psychopharmology Bulletin* 1988, **24**, 629–636.
52. Kokmen E., Smith G.E., Petersen R.C., *et al*. The Short Test of Mental Status: Correlations with Standardised Psychometric Testing. *Archives of Neurology*, 1991, **48**, 725–728.
53. Mattis S. Mental Status Examination for Organic Mental Syndrome in The Elderly Patient. In: L. Bellack and T.D. Karassa (eds). *Geriatric Psychiatry*, 1976, pp. 77–121. Orlando, FL.
54. Wechsler D. *Wechsler Adult Intelligence Scale – Revised 1981*. British Supplement. Psychological Corporation, New York.
55. Jorm A.F., Jacomb P.A. The Informant Questionnaire on Cognitive Decline in the Elderly (IQCODE): Socio-Demographic Correlates, Reliability, Validity and Some Norms. *Psychological Medicine* 1987, **19**, 1015–1022
56. Jorm A.F., Scott R., Cullen J.S., MacKinnon A.J. Performance of the Information Questionnaire on Cognitive Decline in the Elderly (IQCODE) as a Screening Test for Dementia. *Psychological Medicine* 1991, **21**, 785–790.
57. Wechsler D. *Wechsler Memory Scale Revised*, 1987. Psychological Corporation, New York.
58. Morris J.C., Mohs R., Rogers H., *et al*. CERAD Clinical and Neuropsychological Assessment of Alzheimer's Disease. *Psychopharmacology Bulletin* 1988, **24**, 641–651.

59. Welsh K., Butters N., Hughes J., *et al.* Detection of Abnormal Memory Decline in Mild Cases of Alzheimer's Disease Using CERAD Neuropsychological Measures. *Archives of Neurology* 1991, **48**, 278–281.
60. Weintrub S., Mesulan M.N. Mental State Assessment of Young and Elderly Adults in Behavioural Neuropsychology. In: M.N. Mesulan (ed). *Principles of Behavioral Neurology*. Davis, Philadelphia.
61. Warrington E.K. *Camden Memory Tests Manual*, 1996. Psychology Press, Hove.
62. Shay K.A., Duke L.W., Conboy T., *et al.* The Clinical Validity of the Mattis Dementia Rating Scale in Staging Alzheimer's Dementia. *Journal of Geriatric Psychiatry and Neurology* 1991, **4**, 18–25.
63. Gottfries C.G., Brane G., Steen G. A New Rating Scale for Dementia Syndromes. *Gerontology* 1982, **28** (Suppl. 2), 20–31.
64. Nelson H.E., Willison J.R. *National Adult Reading Test (NART) Test Manual*, 2nd edition, 1991. NFER-Nelson, Windsor.
65. Rosen W.G., Mohs R.C., Davis K.L. A New Rating Scale for Alzheimer's Disease. *American Journal of Psychiatry* 1984, **141**, 1356–1364.
66. Kramer-Ginsberg E., Mohs R.C., Aryan N., *et al.* Clinical Predictors of Course for Alzheimer Patients in a Longitudinal Study: A Preliminary Report. *Psychopharmacology Bulletin* 1988, **24**, 458–462.
67. Hughes C.P., Berg L., Danzinger W.L., *et al.* A New Clinical Scale for the Staging of Dementia. *British Journal of Psychiatry* 1982, **140**, 566–572.
68. Berg L. Clinical Dementia Rating (CDR). *Psychopharmacology Bulletin* 1988, **24**, 637–639.
69. Teunisse S., Mayk E., Derix M., Crevel H. Assessing the Severity of Dementia: Patient and Care-giver. *Archives of Neurology* 1991, **48**, 274–277.
70. Hamilton N. Development of a Rating Scale for Primary Depressive Illness. *British Journal of Social and Clinical Psychology* 1967, **6**, 278–296.
71. Williams J.B. A Structured Interview Guide for the Hamilton Depression Rating Scale. *Archives of General Psychiatry* 1988, **45**, 742–747.
72. Yesavage J.A., Blink T.L., Rose T.L., *et al.* Development and Validation of a Geriatric Depression Screening Scale: A Preliminary Report. *Journal of Psychiatric Research* 1983, **17**, 37–49.
73. Zigmond A.F., Snaith R.P. Hospital Anxiety and Depression Scale. *Acta Psychiatrica Scandinavica* 1983, **67**, 361–370.
74. Knopman D.S., Knapp M.J., Grason S.I., Davis C.S. The Clinical Interview-Based Impression (CIBI): A Clinician's Global Change Rating Scale in Alzheimer's Disease. *Neurology* 1994, **44**, 2315–2321.
75. Crook T.H., Larrabee G.J. Interrelationships among everyday memory tests: stability of factor structure with age. *Neuropsychology* 1988, **2**, 1–12.

Part Three

Psychiatric disorders

8

Anxiety in the elderly

Malcolm H. Lader

INTRODUCTION

Anxiety is an ubiquitous, all-pervasive human emotion which we have all experienced frequently and sometimes severely. It is a normal reaction to threatening events or circumstances in life and in turn it mobilises responses which are designed to ready the body for action, 'fight or flight', and also, on a longer time-scale, to initiate coping responses to restore equilibrium. The normal anxiety response has three major components, namely: the physiological, the behavioural and the cognitive. Early interest in anxiety by Darwin and Cannon and others centred on the physiological responses such as facial expression, adrenaline responses and activation of the hypophyseal–pituitary–adrenal (HPA axis). Next, the behavioural elements were examined both in humans but also in animal models of anxiety (Skinner). Most recently the emphasis has been on cognitive elements (Beck) although this goes back to the ideas of William James in the last century.

We are primarily concerned as professionals with abnormal, morbid and clinical anxiety. This is anxiety which is too severe, too frequent or too all-pervasive for the individual to tolerate and/or which leads to behavioural, social and occupational handicap. Thus, the two main elements are subjective distress and objective impairment: these are the fundamentals of assessment.

From the morass of ill-defined anxiety syndromes has emerged a set of closely linked, even overlapping disorders, best exemplified by the successive refinements of definitions in the Diagnostic and Statistical Manuals of

Psychopharmacology of Cognitive and Psychiatric Disorders in the Elderly. Edited by David Wheatley and David Smith. Published in 1998 by Chapman and Hall, London. ISBN 0 412 82470 1

the American Psychiatric Association (DSMI-IV). These well-defined syndromes are largely seen in patients referred to specialist psychiatrists. In primary care, these disorders are less readily distinguishable, co-morbidity is the rule rather than the exception (e.g. panic disorder plus generalised anxiety disorder) and the clinical picture may evolve over time, often with an increasing admixture of depression. Despite this, it is useful to attempt a primary diagnosis even if management is then tempered by the presence of other symptoms and syndromes. In this chapter, the disorders discussed are generalised anxiety disorder (GAD), panic disorder (PD) with and without phobia (agoraphobia, social phobia or specific phobia), obsessive-compulsive disorder (OCD) and post-traumatic stress disorder (PTSD). No detailed accounts are given; rather general principles of the characteristics of the disorders are set out, the available drugs catalogued and an outline management plan presented.

FEATURES OF ANXIETY IN THE ELDERLY

What is special about anxiety in the elderly? Are they in a placid old age reviewing the past with quiet satisfaction and looking forward to an easy passage out of this world? Or are they beset by worries about their financial status, concern over loneliness, and anxiety over failing capacities and the inevitable end? In fact, surveys suggest that most elderly folk enjoy life and are active almost until the end. Only a minority have a protracted decline and relatively few need long-term care. Anxiety is thus not a major problem in the elderly; adolescence is attended by more anxiety, panics and obsessions. There are of course exceptions, particularly among the indigent elderly. Worries revolve around physical illness with secondary handicaps, financial limitations which may lead to inadequate shelter, food and heat, and concerns over personal safety, particularly on housing estates. All of these problems are compounded by poverty so it is important to make a detailed social and financial assessment.

Aetiology

The anxiety disorders seen in adult life are also encountered in the full-blown form in the elderly [1]. Often personality traits may become exaggerated to the point of handicap. The worrier begins to panic, the meticulous housewife spends all her time cleaning, the shy become socially phobic. Patients with lifelong anxiety disorders find that these persist into old age. Having coped with these symptoms for so long they become stoic or they are often so disillusioned by the lack of efficacy of curative measures provided in primary and secondary care that they cease attending clinics. Others turn to alternative medicine, often spending more than they can afford, or find support in religion.

One fairly common method of presentation in old age is the woman or man who was placed on a tranquilliser years before and has continued to take a moderate dose since then. They realise that this medication seems likely to accompany them to the grave and wonder if it is necessary and/or if it is actually harming them. Sometimes their complacent, pre-scribing GP retires and is replaced by a 'Young Turk' who reviews all tranquilliser users and threatens imminent discontinuation. This discom-bobulates the elderly individual who was unaware that his or her med-ication was a tranquilliser (or an hypnotic) and that dependence may have set in. They seek specialist opinion in a panic and the long history of chronic or relapsing anxiety disorder is apparent.

Neurological conditions may complicate the picture or precipitate the disorder. Anxiety may accompany such neurodegenerative conditions as Alzheimer's disease, Lewy body dementia, Parkinson's disease or follow-ing a stroke. A further confusing complication is that anxiety disorders in the cognitively impaired elderly typically present with dysfunctional behaviour which includes agitation, aggression, shouting and meddle-some and intrusive activities (Chapter 13). Failure to detect this leads to an overemphasis on the behaviour itself, with an incorrect management plan which often relies too heavily on medication to suppress the dis-turbing behaviour. Antipsychotic drugs may be used with the risk of autonomic effects and extrapyramidal signs, and even tardive dyskinesia within a few months. Alternatively, anxiolytic tranquillisers may be given with the risk of inducing a spiral of behavioural toxicity, leading to more and more sedation with the release of unacceptable behaviour. There is also the well-known risk of dependence supervening on long-term use.

DIAGNOSIS

Criteria for GAD, PD and OCD

The most comprehensive, operationally defined and evidence-based cri-teria are those of the DSM-IV, as set out somewhat simplified in Table 8.1.

Differential diagnosis

The exclusion of medical causes of anxiety is a prime consideration in young patients and is even more important in the elderly. Of course, the two can co-exist, an anxiety disorder being secondary to a medical condi-tion. The medical causes of anxiety are listed in Table 8.2.

Some of these are important to bear in mind but others are rarities. The commonest is hyperthyroidism which has many symptoms in common with anxiety, particularly those related to the cardiovascular system, such as palpitations and flushing. Iatrogenic hyperthyroidism may supervene,

Table 8.1 Abbreviated criteria for DSM-IV

Generalised Anxiety Disorder

A. Excessive anxiety and worry (apprehensive expectation), occurring more days than not for at least six months, about a number of events or activities (such as work or school performance).

B. The person finds it difficult to control the worry.

C. The anxiety and worry are associated with three (or more) of the following six symptoms (with at least some symptoms present for more days than not for the past six months):
   (1) restlessness or feeling keyed up or on edge
   (2) being easily fatigued
   (3) difficulty concentrating or mind going blank
   (4) irritability
   (5) muscle tension
   (6) sleep disturbance (difficulty falling or staying asleep, or restless unsatisfying sleep).

D. The focus of the anxiety and worry is not confined to features of an Axis I disorder.

E. The anxiety, worry, or physical symptoms cause clinically significant distress or impairment in social, occupational, or other important areas of functioning.

F. The disturbance is not due to the direct physiological effects of a substance or a general medical condition and does not occur exclusively during a mood disorder, a psychotic disorder, or a pervasive developmental disorder.

Panic Disorder

A. Both (1) and (2):
   (1) recurrent unexpected panic attacks
   (2) at least one of the attacks has been followed by one month (or more) of one (or more) of the following:
       (a) persistent concern about having additional attacks
       (b) worry about the implications of the attack or its consequences (e.g. losing control, having a heart attack, 'going crazy')
       (c) a significant change in behaviour related to the attacks.

B. Absence of agoraphobia.

C. The panic attacks are not due to the direct physiological effects of a substance (e.g. a drug of abuse, a medication) or a general medical condition (e.g. hyperthyroidism).

D. The panic attacks are not better accounted for by another mental disorder.

Obsessive-compulsive Disorder

A. Either obsessions or compulsions:
   Obsessions as defined by (1), (2), (3) and (4):
   (1) recurrent and persistent thoughts, impulses, or images that are experienced, at some time during the disturbance, as intrusive and inappropriate and that cause marked anxiety or distress
   (2) the thoughts, impulses, or images are not simply excessive worries about real-life problems

(3) the person attempts to ignore or suppress such thoughts, impulses, or images or to neutralise them with some other thought or action

(4) the person recognises that the obsessional thoughts, impulses, or images are a product of his or her own mind (not imposed from without as in thought insertion).

Compulsions as defined by (1) and (2):

(1) repetitive behaviours (e.g. hand washing, ordering, checking) or mental acts (e.g. praying, counting, repeating words silently) that the person feels driven to perform in response to an obsession, or according to rules that must be applied rigidly.

(2) the behaviours or mental acts are aimed at preventing or reducing distress or preventing some dreaded event or situation; however, these behaviours or mental acts either are not connected in a realistic way with what they are designed to neutralise or prevent or are clearly excessive.

B. At some point during the course of the disorder, the person has recognised that the obsessions or compulsions are excessive or unreasonable.

C. The obsessions or compulsions cause marked distress, are time consuming, or significantly interfere with the person's normal routine, occupational functioning or usual social activities or relationships.

D. If another Axis I disorder is present, the content of the obsessions or compulsions is not restricted to it.

E. The disturbance is not due to the direct physiological effects of a substance or a general medical condition.

Table 8.2 Organic causes of anxiety

Angina pectoris
Carcinoid syndrome
Cardiac arrhythmias
Cerebral arteriosclerosis
Cerebral neoplasm
Cushing's syndrome
Delirium of various types
Early dementia
Hyperventilation
Hypoglycaemia; hyperinsulinism
Hypo- or hyperparathyroidism
Hypo- or hyperthyroidism
Hypoxic states
Mitral valve prolapse
Myocardial infarction
Partial complex seizures
Phaeochromocytoma
Post-concussion disorders
Pulmonary embolism
Vestibular abnormalities

consequent upon maintaining an elderly person on the same dose of thyroid treatment that was appropriate to their physical state on initial diagnosis years before. Any elderly patient who proffers a history of treated hypothyroidism should have his/her thyroid status reviewed with the aid of biochemical measures such as thyroid-stimulating hormone (TSH). With modern radioimmunoassay techniques, abnormal low levels of TSH, representing oversuppression by exogenous thyroxine, can be determined. Sometimes, an anxiety disorder ushers in frank hyperthyroidism with a delay of 1–2 years. Among other conditions, emphysema may induce symptoms resembling those of PD. Quite often an attack of nocturnal asthma wakes the patient with distressing symptoms which mimic those of PD. Acute anxiety secondary to paroxysmal nocturnal dyspnoea may be the only sign of left ventricular failure shown by the elderly patient.

Iatrogenic causes

Treatments for various conditions may themselves be anxiogenic, for example digitalis or a sympathomimetic agent such as ephedrine. Some old people have been on medication of the same type for many years and obsolescent drugs are often found in their medicine cabinets. The elderly often resort to over-the-counter remedies or rely on folk remedies from their childhood. Some of these substances, such as cough and cold remedies, may be taken regularly or even in excessive amounts. Careful questioning is essential to avoid overlooking such agents which have been taken routinely for so long that the patient fails to volunteer information about them.

Alcohol

Problems related to excessive alcohol use may supervene or increase in the elderly. This can result in anxiety or panics related to alcohol withdrawal – essentially a form of subclinical delirium tremens. The typical pattern is for the patient to develop anxiety attacks in the morning after over-indulgence the night before. Sometimes the patient wakes in a panic.

Caffeine

Caffeine is another agent which can readily induce anxiety and elderly people may become more sensitive to it as they do to other drugs. Insomnia with secondary anxiety about not sleeping ('insomnophobia') is another consequence of caffeinism. Coffee or tea restricted to morning intake may still impact adversely on the following night's sleep, at least in the initial phases. In such circumstances, strict adherence to decaffeinated beverages is required especially if hypnotic medication is to be avoided. The following vignette illustrates this point:

Mr J. de F. was a 75-year-old restaurant proprietor. He noted increasing anxiety attacks characterised by shortness of breath and palpitations. He also developed insomnia taking an hour or two to fall asleep even after an exhausting evening at work. During an average day he drank 10–12 cups of strong Espresso coffee. He was advised to cut down on this intake or to switch to decaffeinated coffee. Soon after his anxiety attacks resolved and his sleep returned to normal. Inadvertently, and without his knowledge, caffeinated coffee was substituted for the decaffeinated, and the anxiety and insomnia returned in full force. Again symptoms resolved when caffeine was removed from his diet.

Depression

Depression in the elderly is a major factor releasing generalised or panic anxiety or activating OCD or PTSD. Although there is some controversy as to the actual incidence and prevalence of major depression in the elderly, the generally accepted incidence of treatable depressive illness is around 10–15%. A confounding factor is the co-presentation with dementia. It is well recognised that depression is common in neurodegenerative diseases, with rates in Parkinson's disease being perhaps more than 50%, and about 30% in dementia of the Alzheimer's type and in multi-infarct dementia. Anxiety and agitation are common in this neuropsychiatric complex and may have several aetiological components. Thus, an agitated patient with Parkinsonism (idiopathic or otherwise) may have poorly controlled dyskinesia, be depressed, have drug toxicity or any combination of these. The presence of appetite and weight loss and sleep disturbance may suggest an underlying depression, but this is often masked by anxiety. Indeed control of the anxiety with an anxiolytic such as diazepam may uncover the depression in unmistakable form. Thus DSM-IV criteria for any putative disorder must always be carefully assessed in the elderly with multiple pathologies.

EPIDEMIOLOGY

Until recently, it was difficult to put a reliable figure on the prevalence, and even more so the incidence, of anxiety disorders of various types in old age. One reason was that diagnostic criteria for currently accepted nosological entities within the rubric of anxiety disorders had not been established; most were grouped as the psychoneuroses. Neither Leighton *et al.* [2] nor Pasamanic *et al.* [3] found any evidence of either an increase or a decrease in the prevalence of psychoneurotic disorders in old age compared with younger age groups. Two surveys in the UK found a prevalence of 10.2% and 11% of psychoneurosis in the elderly.

Another UK study recruited over 1000 elderly people living in Liverpool using a rating scale, the Geriatric Mental State [4,5]. The prevalence of anxiety disorder among females over the age of 65 years was 1.5%, that in males 2.9%. Phobic disorder was the next commonest (1.2%) with hypochondriasis (0.5%) and OCD next (0.20%). Patients were monitored for three years during which time the incidence was just under 0.5% per year. Some patients did remit over this time but many suffered continued symptoms.

In the USA, the most systematic data are available from the Epidemiologic Catchment Area Survey [6]. Over 18 000 subjects were included in the study based on institutional and community surveys of five sites in the USA. At all age groups, GAD was fairly common (up to 5% one-year prevalence rates) but tended to drop over the age of 65 years (2.2%) [6]. The age of onset of the condition tended to be in the 20s and virtually all cases in the over-65s were long-standing. PD showed a marked fall-off in one-year prevalence with age, from around 4% in young adults to less than a tenth of this in the elderly. OCD cases also showed a decline but this was less marked (2% to 0.9%).

PHARMACOKINETICS

This general topic has been reviewed in Chapter 2. The essential point is that the elderly are usually more sensitive to most drugs because of changes in such pharmacokinetic parameters as volume of distribution, hepatic metabolism and renal clearance rate [7]. Sedatives, tranquillisers and antidepressants are examples of drugs to which this generalisation applies. Furthermore, the elderly may become more sensitive pharmacodynamically because of changes in receptors and in receptor–effector coupling.

In practical terms the elderly may be more sensitive overall by a factor of two or three, or even more in the aged and multiply impaired. As drugs act longer, less frequent dosing may be feasible. It is usual to initiate drug treatment at half-dosage or even less and to push the dose slowly: 'Start low and go slow'. Some elderly patients, however, may need full doses and appear to tolerate them, thus it is important to try and achieve full dosage if the patient is comfortable with this regimen.

AVAILABLE TREATMENTS

In the late 19th and early 20th centuries, the most extensively used drugs were the bromides. Unfortunately, their adverse effects were slow to become appreciated, toxic delirium being the most serious. This was a particular problem in the elderly because their age-related decline in renal function resulted in an accumulation of bromide in the body. Phenobarbitone was also commonly used; other barbiturates were introduced to help manage anxiety: these included amylobarbitone and quinalbarbitone. These drugs were found to have a high likelihood of inducing dependence, toxicity such as confusion and delirium in high doses and the danger of overdose, accidental or deliberate. All these compounds are now obsolete but one still encounters the occasional elderly patient who is still taking a barbiturate regularly after many years.

In the 1950s attempts were made to develop a better anxiolytic. The first candidate was meprobamate which enjoyed a brief vogue until it was found to possess most, if not all, of the drawbacks of the barbiturates. It was fairly rapidly superseded by the benzodiazepines, the first one of which, chlordiazepoxide, was introduced in 1959. Many others have followed. Of these, alprazolam has the additional indication in the USA of PD.

Antidepressant drugs have also been evaluated as anxiolytics. The earliest examples are the monoamine oxidase inhibitors (MAOIs) which were used extensively and often uncritically in 'atypical depression', a vague description of depressed patients who often suffered as well from phobic anxiety and panics. More recently, imipramine and clomipramine, both tricyclic antidepressants (TCA), have been evaluated in PD and the latter particularly in OCD. Efficacy has been established unequivocally but these tricyclic drugs are often poorly tolerated in the elderly. Over the past decade the selective serotonin reuptake inhibitor (SSRI) antidepressants have been tested in PD patients. All appear fairly effective in these conditions and one, paroxetine, has been licensed for those indications in the UK and in Canada. By contrast efficacy in OCD is less well established.

Current choices

Detailed accounts of anxiolytic and antidepressant medications are available in standard textbooks [8]. The following brief overview concentrates on their profile in the elderly [9].

Benzodiazepines

For the past three decades, this class of drugs has been used, particularly in primary care, as the main treatment for anxiety and related disorders. They bind to the benzodiazepine–GABA–chloride ionophore receptor complex. These structures are widespread throughout the brain, particularly in the cerebral and cerebellar cortices. The benzodiazepines induce anxiolysis, sedation, sleep and muscle relaxation, and most have an anticonvulsive effect. Autonomic function is but little affected. They can produce profound impairments of psychomotor ability to the point of ataxia and cognitive function to the point of amnesia [10].

Many but not all are metabolised slowly in the elderly, so that particular toxicity problems may arise. Many of these have been reviewed in

Chapter 3. The most common subjective side-effects are fatigue, tiredness, drowsiness, tremor, muscle weakness, dysarthria and ataxia. Confusion and depression may supervene at higher doses. Occasionally paradoxical anxiety, aggression or mania is induced. Particular problems in the elderly to which attention has been drawn are the increased risk of falls and hip fractures and the hazard of road accidents [11].

Benzodiazepines are generally fairly safe in the elderly who are physically ill, although respiratory function can be depressed further in patients with chronic obstructive lung disease. The resulting anoxaemia can result in a confusional state. As in younger patients, habituation, dependence and withdrawal syndromes can occur in the elderly and be troublesome. By simple chronology, the elderly are more likely to be long-term users of benzodiazepines than younger subjects. Generally, the widespread and sometimes indiscriminate use of benzodiazepines in the institutionalised elderly is a major cause of significant morbidity and probably mortality [12].

Buspirone

This novel anxiolytic was introduced several years ago. It is chemically distinct from the benzodiazepines and it acts on serotonin not GABA mechanisms. It is fairly effective but has the drawback of a slow progression of action, in contrast to the rapid and obvious effect of the benzodiazepines. Side-effects include nausea, dizziness, headache and fatigue, and are often quite marked about an hour after each dose. Psychomotor and cognitive impairment is minimal, as is dependence potential and abuse liability. Consequently, it may be particularly useful in the elderly, particularly those intolerant of a benzodiazepine.

Antipsychotics

In some countries, but not commonly now in the UK, antipsychotic medication in low dose is prescribed as an anti-anxiety therapy. Unfortunately, extrapyramidal effects such as akathisia and Parkinsonism may occur even at low dosage; the elderly are notably more susceptible to these unwanted effects. Also, tardive dyskinesia poses a risk in long-term treatment even at low dose. Neuroleptic malignant syndrome (NMS), or at least a transient variant, may be more common in the elderly than appreciated (Chapter 3). Acute confusion with rigidity, a high white cell count, rising creatinine kinase and pyrexia are highly indicative of this potentially fatal syndrome. Early signs of NMS often include anxiety which may mislead the clinician. Management includes the immediate cessation of the neuroleptic and measures to reduce core temperature. Drugs such as dantrolene or bromocriptine are usually unnecessary.

Postural hypotension is another problem in the elderly, with the age-related impairment of maintaining blood pressure being exaggerated by the alpha-blocking effect of many neuroleptics. This may lead to falls and subsequent fractures.

Antihistamines

Diphenhydramine and hydroxyzine are sometimes prescribed for the anxious elderly individual. Antihistamines have concomitant anticholinergic effects such as dry mouth, blurred vision, confusion and severe (sometimes obstructive) constipation, to which the elderly are especially prone. Sedation is also quite marked and confusion and disorientation may occur. While it may be true that dependence does not develop, it is clear that in a few elderly doses may increase slowly. This results in increasing toxicity over time.

Beta-blockers

These drugs are often prescribed for patients with agoraphobia or social phobias. They reduce such symptoms as palpitations, tremor and gastrointestinal upset but may not assuage subjective anxiety. Some patients find them useful, others report only limited relief. The hypotensive effect of these drugs and the sense of tiredness they engender limits their use in the elderly.

Antidepressant drugs

Various groups of antidepressants are being resorted to increasingly in the management of the range of anxiety disorders. Some are already licensed for the indication of anxiety within the context of a depressive illness, others for mixed anxiety-depressive states. Some antidepressants, clomipramine and SSRIs to a lesser extent, are effective in OCD. PD is another indication which is under evaluation: SSRIs are proving quite effective, and paroxetine has been licensed for this indication in the UK. However, efficacy data in the elderly are lacking. Phobic anxiety has been a traditional target for the MAOIs. For example, several recent studies attest to the efficacy of MAOIs in social phobia. Again, data in the elderly are not extant.

Among the antidepressants, the TCAs are often poorly tolerated in the elderly because of sedation and autonomic side-effects such as postural hypotension, dry mouth and constipation [13]. The traditional MAOIs are also poorly tolerated in the elderly, severe postural hypotension limiting the dosage attainable. The SSRIs and the RIMA (reversible inhibitor of monoamineoxidase A) moclobemide are generally preferable, although the long elimination time of norfluoxetine makes fluoxetine a poor choice in the elderly. Paroxetine, initially at 10 mg, appears to be an effective choice for the treatment of depression in the elderly, especially those with anxiety. The SSRIs tend to have complex metabolic patterns involving one or more cytochrome systems so the co-prescription of other medications must be undertaken with the utmost care and circumspection.

Venlafaxine is a recently introduced drug blocking both noradrenaline and serotonin reuptake systems. Many psychiatrists regard it as effective in cases of depression that have proven refractory to other agents, but it can be prescribed for any depressed patient. It is reasonably well tolerated in the elderly.

Electroconvulsive therapy (ECT)

Although ECT is not specifically indicated for anxiety, agitated elderly patients with depression not uncommonly will require this treatment. Often, these frail patients cannot tolerate chemotherapy or have not responded. Contrary to lay opinions, ECT is actually safe and often effective. For patients with Parkinson's disease and depression, ECT will benefit both the mood and motor symptoms and should be considered at an earlier stage than might otherwise pertain. The presence of a co-morbid dementia is *not* a contraindication to ECT and there continues to be *no* evidence that demonstrates that ECT causes further brain damage.

PRACTICAL DRUG MANAGEMENT

Only broad guidelines can be given here and these reflect my current personal preferences. The essential steps in treatment are:

1. Explanation, reassurance and discussion with both the patient and his/her carers.
2. The abnormal symptoms and behaviour must be counteracted and brought back under the patient's control. This includes suppression of obsessive thoughts and compulsive rituals, lessening of panics in terms of both frequency and severity, and amelioration of anticipatory, free-floating anxiety. This is applicable to the range of disorders from GAD to PTSD.
3. While these symptoms are maintained at a low and tolerable level, appropriate anxiety management and/or cognitive behaviour therapy (CBT) is instituted to alter behaviour, e.g. agoraphobic avoidance and to change cognitions.
4. The drugs are slowly withdrawn.

Because the duration of this type of treatment strategy encompasses months rather than weeks, benzodiazepines are not suitable medications. This is especially so because effective dosages tend to be high and therefore more likely to induce dependence. The only role for these drugs is as short-term (less than two weeks) therapy for the rapid relief of intolerable anxiety during an acute exacerbation.

Currently, SSRI antidepressants seem to be the treatment of choice. Of these, paroxetine is licensed for panic disorder in some countries (including the UK) and it and fluoxetine are licensed in some countries for OCD. In general, the doses needed to control OCD and suppress panics are substantially higher than the antidepressant doses. As SSRIs are *anxiogenic* during the first week or so of administration, half-doses are essential initially, and the patient must be warned of this side-effect. Then the dosage can be titrated upwards fairly slowly as necessary. Although not licensed for this indication, it is my experience that they are often effective in GAD as well, particularly those patients with co-morbid depression or an admixture of 'reactive' depression. The main side-effects of the SSRIs in the elderly are headache, dizziness and nausea, but these are usually markedly dose-dependent and tolerance is exhibited. Complaints of sexual dysfunction are not usually observed.

The subsequent psychological treatment must be tailored to the individual symptomatic/behavioural needs of the patient. Such treatment must be expert: training in non-focused techniques, such as relaxation, may not be helpful and some patients may become more panicky as they 'relax'. The patient must be prepared to invest time and energy in cooperating in the treatment, which need not be prolonged. More traditional psychotherapies *may* be useful in some patients with complex and abnormal personal relationships or deeply rooted and symbolic symptom-reactions.

CONCLUSIONS

As in younger populations, anxiety in the elderly is a non-specific marker for distress as well as disease. Moreover, neurodegenerative changes in the elderly further complicate this picture. The elderly often present with multiple illnesses and are taking many different medications; therefore simply adding on the diagnosis of 'anxiety' and prescribing a tranquilliser will invariably worsen the situation. Care must always be taken to obtain a detailed history, with collateral witnesses, and to conduct a careful examination of both physical and mental states. The possibility of the anxiety or agitation being a presentation of drug toxicity should be considered early. Only when physical causes have been eliminated or at least stabilised should psychiatric causes be explored.

Depression and dementia remain the most common causes of anxiety in the elderly. As with antidepressants, anxiolytics should be chosen with care and used as part of a planned management package. Emergent toxicity should always be anticipated and the patient should be reviewed frequently. Supportive therapies are always helpful and can help establish realistic therapeutic goals and optimise compliance. While it is true that the world is a more threatening place for the elderly, it is equally true that the majority of old people are not frightened and cope extremely well. Prejudice and stereotyping must be avoided and each case assessed individually and thoroughly. This may take more time but the physician must avoid adding to the burden the patient has to bear. Becoming anxious must never be dismissed as an inevitable and untreatable feature of ageing.

REFERENCES

1. Sheikh, J.I. and Swales, P.J. (1994) Clinical features of anxiety disorders. In *Principles and Practice of Geriatric Psychiatry* (eds J.R.M. Copeland, M.T. Abou-Saleh and D.G. Blazer), John Wiley, Chichester, pp. 725–9.
2. Leighton, D.C., Harding, D.S. and Macklin, D.B. (1963) *The Character of Danger*, Basic Books, New York.
3. Pasamanic, B., Roberts, D.W., Limkau, P.W. and Krueger, D.B. (1959) A survey of mental disease in an urban population: prevalence by race and income. In *Epidemiology of Mental Disorder* (ed. B. Pasamanic), American Association for the Advancement of Science, Washington, DC, pp. 183–202.
4. Copeland, J.R.M., Dewey, M.E., Wood, H. *et al.* (1987) Range of mental illness among elderly in the community: prevalence in Liverpool using GMS-AGE-CAT package. *British Journal of Psychiatry*, **150**, 815–23.
5. Larkin, B.A., Copeland, J.R.M. Dewey, M.L. *et al.* (1992) The natural history of neurotic disorders in an elderly urban population: findings from Liverpool longitudinal study of continuing health in the community. *British Journal of Psychiatry*, **160**, 681–6.
6. Blazer, D.G. (1994) Epidemiology. In *Principles and Practice of Geriatric Psychiatry* (eds J.R.M. Copeland, M.T. Abou-Saleh and D.G. Blazer), John Wiley, Chichester, pp. 715–18.
7. Lader, M. (1991) Neuropharmacology and pharmacokinetics of psychotropic drugs in old age, in *Psychiatric Disorders in America* (eds L.N. Robins and D.A. Regier), Free Press, New York, pp. 79–82.
8. Lader, M. and Herrington, R. (1996) *Biological Treatments in Psychiatry*, 2nd Edition, Oxford University Press, Oxford.
9. Dia, A.R., Ranga, K. and Krishnan, R. (1994) Psychopharmacological treatment of anxiety disorders. In *Principles and Practice of Geriatric Psychiatry* (eds J.R.M. Copeland, M.T. Abou-Saleh and D.G. Blazer), John Wiley, Chichester, pp. 741–9.
10. Ancill, R.J., Embury, G.D., MacEwan, G.W. *et al.* (1987) Lorazepam in the elderly – a retrospective study of the side-effects in 20 patients. *Journal of Psychopharmacology*, **2**, 126–7.
11. Ray, W.A., Griffin, M.R. and Downey, W. (1989) Benzodiazepines of long and short elimination half-life and the risk of hip fracture. *Journal of the American Medical Association*, **262**, 3303–7.
12. Larson, E.B., Kukull, W.A., Buchner, D. *et al.* (1987) Adverse drug reactions associated with global cognitive impairment in elderly persons. *Annals of Internal Medicine*, **107**, 169–73.
13. Katona, C. (1993) The management of depression in old age. In *Depression in Old Age* (ed. C. Katona), John Wiley, Chichester, pp. 105.

9

Treatment of depression in old age

Stuart A. Montgomery and Anita Kotak

INTRODUCTION

In recent years it has been observed that the incidence of depression may be increasing and attention has been focused on the implications for health care systems. The extent of any general increase is the subject of some dispute as the comparisons of prevalence rates are likely to have been biased by the methods of data collection. Nevertheless, one undoubted factor in a rise in depression is the increasing numbers of the aged who, in all developed countries, have increased not only in absolute numbers as longevity becomes more common but also as a proportion of the general population.

The problem of provision of care for this growing elderly population is a matter of concern for the immediate future and is exacerbated by the concurrent decline in the size of the economically active population. The elderly are major users of health services, occupying half the medical beds and nearly half the psychiatric beds in hospitals in the UK. Approximately half of all prescribed medications in the UK are for the elderly, defined as those aged over 65 years of age, although they make up only 18% of the population. Clearly the elderly have a high incidence of both physical and psychiatric illness and an increase in health care spending for this age group is inevitable. Nevertheless there are a number of strategies available to reduce the unnecessary utilisation of health care resources and at the same time to improve their quality of life.

Psychopharmacology of Cognitive and Psychiatric Disorders in the Elderly. Edited by David Wheatley and David Smith. Published in 1998 by Chapman and Hall, London. ISBN 0 412 82470 1

It is important that depression in the elderly should be detected because of the well-recognised risk of suicide associated with the disorder, a risk that may be higher among elderly patients [1]. It is also reported that depression can have an influence in both causing psychological illness and in slowing down recovery from physical illnesses in elderly patients [2,3]. The undertreatment of depression in the elderly should therefore be a matter of concern. Community studies have estimated that as few as 4% of elderly depressed patients receive appropriate treatment and the rate is not a great deal higher among primary care attenders [4]. Of those treated with tricyclic antidepressants (TCA), less than 20% receive adequate doses in primary care.

Depression is common in the elderly and depressive symptomatology is reported to occur in around 15% of a clinical sample aged 65 years and over [5]. The prevalence of depression in the elderly is probably even higher than in the general population though it may often be underestimated. This is to some extent because of the still quite prevalent attitude, even among physicians, of resignation which regards old age as a time of inevitable decline, incapacity and gloom. The pessimism and apathy so frequently seen in old people are taken to be a normal consequence of ageing, but such despondency may, and frequently does, represent an undetected treatable depressive illness.

PROBLEMS OF DIAGNOSIS

Depression in the elderly may be missed for a variety of reasons. These include failure by the physician to recognise the illness or, if it is recognised, a failure to acknowledge the condition and the need for vigorous treatment. Patients also often lack understanding and may not recognise their depressive symptoms as appropriate for medical intervention.

Somatic presentation

Late-life depression sometimes has a somewhat atypical appearance which may lead to the diagnosis being missed [5]. The elderly depressed patient, unlike younger patients, may not complain primarily of depressed mood and the treating physicians may need a high index of suspicion to detect it. Depression in the elderly tends to manifest itself with somatic symptoms, and the patient frequently complains of specific or non-specific pains, discomforts or general unwellness. This is possibly a consequence of the attitude that old age is primarily a time of regret, disappointment and loss, a condition to be borne with fortitude which leads the elderly depressed patient to focus his or her disorder on physical symptoms.

These somatic complaints may become very insistent, even reaching hypochondriacal proportions. Nevertheless, the physician may not identify the covert depression because with the risk of physical illness being so high in the elderly, a physical cause is sought. There may sometimes be considerable delay before the patient's illness is recognised as having a psychological basis.

Medical illness

Some physical illness, which is far more prevalent in the older age group, may mask or mimic depressive symptomatology [6]. For example, neoplasia may manifest itself in the early stages with behavioural changes. Metabolic disturbances such as abnormalities of serum glucose, potassium, calcium and hepatic dysfunction, as well as endocrine disturbances and infectious disease, can all lead to apathy, lack of activity and anorexia. Such symptoms are more difficult to assess in the elderly than in younger patients because the variation between elderly individuals in level of normal functioning is very much wider.

Much depression in the elderly is also probably overlooked because of a bias towards the diagnosis of dementia. Confusion and memory impairment are common features of many illnesses in old people including depression and may be misdiagnosed as dementia. In many cases when the depression is treated the 'pseudo dementia' disappears. On the other hand the prevalence of depression is reported to be elevated in patients with Alzheimer's disease and while it may be difficult to assess in these patients, treatment is important as it can improve cognitive function as well as alleviate the depression.

RESPONSE TO TREATMENT

Our knowledge about the relative efficacy of antidepressants in the treatment of depression in the elderly has been restricted to some extent by the exclusion of elderly patients from the clinical efficacy trials of antidepressants. The large clinical trial programmes carried out with more recently introduced antidepressants, however, have included sufficient patients across the age spectrum to be able to make the assessment that antidepressants are effective in both younger and older patients.

Earlier studies suggested there might be some differences between elderly and younger patients and that the elderly might tend to be more treatment resistant or to show a slower response to treatment [7]. More recent studies have shown that a good response to antidepressants is obtained in the elderly in the acute treatment of depression. An early study that compared elderly and younger patients in different age cohorts found a poorer response in the elderly using a cutoff of 55 years, but when the patients aged over 65 years were examined a response similar to that in the younger patients was seen [8]. An analysis of response rates in the elderly carried out in the USA found a rate of response similar to that expected in the general depressed population among the younger elderly patients although in those aged over 80 years the response rate was lower [9]. There is certainly no consistent evidence that would support the concept that elderly depression does not respond to antidepressant treatment. Depression in late life is, however, a chronic or relapsing condition and close followup is required [10].

COMPLICATIONS OF TREATMENT

Treatment with antidepressants is complicated by physiological factors related directly to the ageing process by the frequent presence of comorbid physical illness and by compliance difficulties due to forgetfulness, poor understanding or an inability to tolerate side-effects.

The process of ageing has a profound effect on the disposition of drugs (Chapter 2). End organ sensitivity and decreased receptor responsiveness can lead to changes in pharmacodynamics and a higher side-effects burden may result. Reduced renal and hepatic function is more likely in the elderly and will affect drug clearance and the plasma concentrations of the drug achieved. The effect is seen in the interindividual variability in the steady-state plasma concentrations which are produced by the same dose of a drug, being much greater with increased age.

The possibility of drug interactions is increased during the treatment of elderly patients because of the likelihood of concomitant physical illness for which the patient is receiving medication. These adverse reactions, which are three times as likely in the elderly as in young patients under the age of 30 years, are a major cause of morbidity and mortality in the elderly. The selection of an antidepressant for the elderly patient has to take this increased risk from polypharmacy into consideration.

EFFICACY

There have been relatively few specific studies examining the efficacy of antidepressants in the elderly and comparisons across studies are made difficult because of the varying definitions of 'elderly' and because of the high and variable rates of discontinuations from the study [11]. In general, however, the antidepressant effect seems to be in accord with studies in younger populations.

New antidepressants

The selective serotonin reuptake inhibitors (SSRIs) have been shown to be effective antidepressants [12] and concerns expressed about the possibility that they might not be as effective as tricyclic antidepressants (TCAs) in severe depression do not appear to have been justified. In the clinical trial programmes with these drugs, the many placebo controlled studies included a reference TCA control group, and the databases are sufficiently large to be able to estimate relative efficacy. These analyses have shown that SSRIs generally are of the same order of efficacy as the TCAs in the general depressed population.

Pooled analyses of the data also indicate that there may be an advantage in severe depression for SSRIs compared with the TCA imipramine [13]. There are few direct comparisons of one SSRI with another so that it would not be possible to draw any conclusions on the respective merits of these drugs which do have some variation in their pharmacological profile; however, the studies indicate a similar therapeutic benefit between the different compounds.

Citalopram

The studies of citalopram took account of the complicated clinical picture presented sometimes by the elderly and included a population of patients with dementia and depression [14,15]. On a number of measures of depression and emotional disturbance which included depressed mood, citalopram was seen to be effective compared with placebo though it did not have an effect in improving dementia. A second study addressed elderly patients with depression, some of whom had dementia, and a significant advantage of citalopram compared with placebo was demonstrated.

Citalopram has also been investigated in depression associated with physical illness in two studies of post-stroke depression and was again found to be effective in alleviating the depression.

Fluvoxamine

This drug was shown to be as effective as imipramine and better than placebo in a small study of a relatively young elderly group and, in comparator studies which showed the same order of effect size to the expected in the young depressed population, to have a similar level of efficacy to dothiepin and to mianserin [16–18].

Fluoxetine

This drug was reported to be better than placebo in a large study in the elderly [19] and to be of the same order of efficacy as reference TCAs, though the effect size was quite modest [20,21]. In a small study in the elderly, fluoxetine was found to have similar efficacy to trazodone [22].

Paroxetine

This drug has been shown to be as effective as doxepin in a relatively large study in the elderly and in smaller studies has been reported to be as effective as amitriptyline, clomipramine, mianserin and fluoxetine [23–27]. A metanalysis carried out on comparator studies in the elderly showed a significant advantage for paroxetine [28].

Sertraline

This drug has been reported to be of the same order of efficacy as amitriptyline in a comparator study, but this study suffered from a particularly high attrition rate [29].

Venlafaxine

This selective inhibitor with a double action on the reuptake of serotonin and noradrenaline is an effective antidepressant which may well have particular efficacy in severely depressed inpatients when used in higher doses [30]. It seems to have a rapid onset of action if doses are escalated rapidly in the first week [31].

Mirtazepine

Mirtazepine, a α_2 antagonist and specific serotonin 2 and 3 antagonist, seems to have a double action on both noradrenaline and serotonin that is mediated through S_{1A} receptors. The S_2 and S_3 antagonism reduces the serotonin side-effects substantially and greatly improves tolerability. It seems from comparator studies to be effective and well tolerated in the elderly [32].

LONG-TERM TREATMENT

The principles behind long-term treatment in the elderly are similar to those in younger patients. After acute symptomatic response, antidepressants need to be taken for a period of continuation treatment to ensure that the response stabilises. The length of this continuation period is normally thought to last some four to six months. There have been very few studies specifically in an elderly population but it is possible that this continuation period needs to be longer in the elderly.

The TCAs, nortriptyline and dothiepin, have both been studied in an elderly depressed population and the results are disappointing [33,34]. The study of nortriptyline was well designed, placebo and reference controlled and used plasma level monitoring, even though a low mean dose

was used. Nortriptyline was not found to differ from placebo in maintenance or prophylactic treatment, and to be worse than phenelzine which
was itself effective. Dothiepin in a modest dose seemed to be effective in
the continuation treatment phase and then to lose efficacy in the rest of
the two-year study. It would seem that the finding that full doses of antidepressants are needed for prophylaxis in younger patients is probably
also true in the elderly. For this reason it is important that well-tolerated
and effective antidepressants are used in treating old age depression in
both the short and long-term.

The findings on efficacy in elderly depressed patients with the different antidepressants are consistent and do not give rise to any suspicion
that antidepressants that are effective in the general age range of
depressed patients will not also be effective in the elderly. What is of
more interest in the selection of an antidepressant is therefore the tolerability profile of the antidepressant.

THE SIDE-EFFECT BURDEN

Problems of the TCAs

One of the important reasons for undertreatment of depression has been
identified as the prescription of poorly tolerated antidepressants which
lead to premature discontinuation of treatment. This is a particular problem with the traditional TCAs which are well known to be associated
with a high level of unwanted effects [35]. These drugs have a wide
range of pharmacological effects in addition to those which bring about
their therapeutic action. Patients find the anticholinergic, adrenergic and
histaminergic effects of these antidepressants difficult to tolerate and
often withdraw from treatment because of them.

In elderly patients the problem is particularly acute. The TCAs have
marked cardiotoxic effects, including negative ionotropism and a quinidine-like effect which can lead to bundle branch patterns, QRS widening
and even heart block and arrhythmias. Elderly patients who may be at
risk of compromised cardiac function may suffer worsening of cardiovascular disease during treatment with these drugs.

Some side-effects may be of less concern in younger patients but cause
problems in the elderly because of concomitant physical problems.
Confusion may be increased in patients who are suffering from mild
dementia. Bodyweight gain, which frequently accompanies treatment
with TCAs, can obviously be detrimental to those with congestive heart
failure, diabetes or arthritis. Some TCAs are particularly sedative which
can be a problem in all age groups but in the elderly may interfere with
cognitive function which is itself often compromised in the elderly [36]. It
has been reported that the risk of injury in car accidents is twice as high

in individuals aged over 65 years taking TCAs, compared with age-matched controls not receiving TCAs.

The TCAs have a potent effect in blocking α_1 adrenergic receptors and this may exacerbate postural hypotension in elderly depressed patients. What might well be regarded as an inconvenience for younger, physically healthy patients can have serious consequences in the elderly who are more prone to serious falls and fractures [37].

Age-related changes in drug handling in elderly patients are an important problem with TCA treatment: impaired hepatic function affects clearance, age-related reduction in protein synthesis can lead to an increase in drug plasma levels, etc. Some of the undesirable effects can be reduced by giving a lower than standard dose in the elderly but this will not overcome the problem of the unpredictable interindividual variability in plasma levels achieved. This is a particular issue as the therapeutic range is relatively narrow with some of the older TCAs.

Side-effects and new antidepressants

More recent antidepressants have been developed on the basis of having a pharmacological profile that is more selective with the aim of reducing the unwanted side-effects associated with the TCAs. They have not fulfilled the hope that they would prove to be more effective than the reference TCAs, but they have been shown to be of the same order of efficacy with the advantage of an improved side-effect and safety profile. This is an important factor in the choice of treatment for the elderly because of the increased sensitivity of this group to adverse drug reactions. It is unlikely that any effective active drug will be entirely free of unwanted effects but several of the newer antidepressants have very benign side-effect profiles and this would make them a preferred choice of treatment for elderly depressed patients. The improved tolerability helps with compliance with treatment and some metanalyses have reported a lower number of discontinuations from side-effects with the SSRIs compared with TCAs [38,39].

SSRIs

The selective action of the SSRIs on the serotoninergic pathway brings about the characteristic adverse effects expected from this pharmacological profile. These include gastrointestinal symptoms and sometimes the appearance of anxiety or an exacerbation of anxiety in some patients. The SSRIs are generally non-sedative drugs, which is an advantage in elderly patients, but there are some differences in this respect between compounds, with paroxetine reported to be associated with more drowsiness than other SSRIs. In general, they have a neutral psychomotor effect, do not appear to cause cognitive impairment and may even have some action in improving cognitive function. Some of the side-effects are dose related, for example nausea, which seems to be more of a problem with fluvoxamine.

The appearance of anxiety early in treatment is thought to be more likely with fluoxetine and this might appear to be a disadvantage in the elderly where depression frequently presents with agitation. Placebo-controlled studies have shown that the SSRIs have an advantage compared with reference TCAs in ameliorating the symptoms of anxiety during acute treatment [40].

The SSRIs have little affinity for α_1 receptors and are therefore less likely to cause postural hypotension than the older TCAs; the lack of anticholinergic effects makes them a much more readily tolerated treatment.

Nefazodone

Nefazodone lacks the adverse effects on sexual function which are associated with the SSRIs but in other respects the side-effect profile is very similar.

Venlafaxine

Venlafaxine has the advantage of a faster onset of action seen in severely depressed hospitalised patients but it is associated with a heavier side-effect profile [30,41]. Any therapeutic advantage of venlafaxine over other antidepressants appears to depend on the rapid escalation of dose early in treatment, but this results in a greater side-effect burden than some of the other recent drugs. The likelihood of side-effects may be particularly burdensome for elderly patients.

Mirtazepine

One of the more recently introduced antidepressants, mirtazepine has been shown to be as effective as reference TCAs, more effective than one SSRI [32,42,43] and to have a very low frequency of side-effects. This low level of side-effects was reflected in an advantage for mirtazepine in comparison to TCAs in producing a lower rate of discontinuations from treatment due to side-effects. The main side-effect reported was sedation, and this was mainly mild and of short duration. One complication of treatment with mirtazepine in elderly patients is that at low doses this antidepressant has more sedative action than at higher doses. If elderly patients are given lower doses in order to allow for the possibility of age-related changes in drug handling they may be exposed to the disadvantage of excess drowsiness and should be followed up to check for this side-effect.

SAFETY ISSUES

Safety is an important consideration particularly in overdose because, in addition to the risk of deliberate overdose present with depression, in the elderly there is a risk of overdose happening because of forgetfulness.

The newer antidepressants represent an important advance over the TCAs as regards cardiac effects. The use of the TCAs in the elderly, in whom there is a risk of undetected cardiac problems, has been limited because of the significant effects on the electrocardiograph (ECG) observed with these drugs even at therapeutic doses [44]. The SSRIs, venlafaxine and mirtazepine overall cause fewer conduction effects and in the clinical development programmes have had a safer profile in relation to cardiac effects than the reference TCAs. The relatively benign adverse event profile in the general age range samples of depressed patients with the newer antidepressants also appears to hold in the elderly patients, as analyses that have separated out the elderly from younger patients have shown. There are, however, case reports of cardiac effects with the SSRIs, including reports of bradycardia and dysrhythmias in elderly patients with preexisting heart disease [45–48].

Overall the relative lack of cardiotoxic effects may contribute to the newer drugs being safer in overdose than the older TCAs. The indices of toxicity that can be drawn up from the reports of deaths from overdose with antidepressants show a high rate of death from overdose with TCAs, particularly dothiepin and amitriptyline, and a consistently low rate with the newer antidepressants [49].

Drug interactions, which are a risk in the elderly because of the likelihood of polypharmacy, include the potentiation of the effects of diuretics or beta-blockers by TCAs because of their activity at α_1 adrenoceptors. The TCAs can also augment the CNS depressant effects of alcohol and of benzodiazepines.

The neuroleptic malignant syndrome, which might well be the same as the serotonin syndrome, is a potentially fatal consequence of a drug interaction. The elderly may be more prone to this reaction both because of the inherent variability of enzyme activity in the elderly and because of the increased number of drugs taken by them, with the greater likelihood of reactions. A variety of drugs are implicated. The phenomenon was first reported with high doses of lithium and neuroleptics but more recently deaths have been reported with monoamine oxidase inhibitors and SSRIs. The combination of clomipramine and tranylcypramine has been reported to be associated with a number of deaths. Deaths have also been reported with fluoxetine in combination with phenelzine and it is now recommended that a sufficient interval of two to three weeks is left to allow a washout of MAOI before introducing a SSRI. Because of the prolonged half-life of the active metabolite of fluoxetine, a five-week washout is required with this antidepressant before instituting therapy with a MAOI.

Pharmacokinetics

Changes in pharmacokinetics would be expected in the elderly and this has been examined with the newer antidepressants (Chapter 2). Age-related change in clearance has been reported with some SSRIs but not with all. For example, clearance of citalopram and paroxetine is reduced in elderly patients compared with that in younger patients [50,51]. Steady-state plasma concentrations of citalopram were higher in the elderly, with the same dose, than in younger patients, and the half-life of paroxetine was increased in the elderly though there was considerable overlap. An increase in fluoxetine plasma concentrations was observed in the elderly compared with younger patients, and there were some differences between the elderly and younger subjects in the investigations of sertraline, although these were small [52,53]. In most of the investigations there is considerable overlap between the elderly and younger subjects. Age-related changes in drug handling were least apparent with fluvoxamine [54]. Caution nevertheless dictates that lower doses are used in the elderly than in younger patients, if only because of the increased risk of physical disease which may also affect drug disposition.

The likelihood that elderly patients will be taking more than one medication, in addition to any treatment for depression focuses attention on a potential problem of treatment with SSRIs. These antidepressants inhibit specific cytochrome P450 enzymes involved in the elimination of drugs and pharmacokinetic interactions can arise when SSRIs are prescribed concomitantly with other drugs that are metabolised via the cytochrome P450 system. Inhibition of the cytochrome P450 system can produce reduced clearance of a range of drugs in common use, such as TCAs and phenothiazines, as well as anticoagulants and some antiarrhythmics.

There are differences between the SSRIs in the extent to which they affect the cytochrome P450 system, citalopram being the least potent in this respect [55]. Fluvoxamine has little activity on P450IID6 but there are some reports of interreactions on the P450IIIA system.

SELECTING AN ANTIDEPRESSANT FOR ELDERLY DEPRESSION

The ideal antidepressant to be used in an old age population is one that is clearly effective at doses that are well tolerated. Those antidepressants that have a high side-effects burden, or are only effective at high doses which are difficult to tolerate, should probably not be used as first line treatment in the elderly. TCAs in general are used at doses for which efficacy has not been demonstrated, and their potential efficacy is compromised by the difficulty of persuading depressed patients to tolerate the side-effects of effective doses. In the elderly the side-effects burden is more difficult to tolerate and these patients are more vulnerable to cardiac complications and fractures from falling. For these reasons TCAs are best avoided in treating depression in old age.

Among the effective, well-tolerated and widely available antidepressants there are a range of SSRIs (fluoxetine, fluvoxamine, paroxetine, sertraline and citalopram), and even newer antidepressants, such as nefazadone or mirtazepine, to choose from. Safety and tolerability are essential as long as this is compatible with giving the appropriate dose to ensure that response is achieved. Of those antidepressants not yet as widely available, tianeptine, milnacipran and reboxetine all show good efficacy and tolerability and these should widen the range of treatments which are useful in the elderly.

REFERENCES

1. Conwell, Y. and Brent, D. (1995) Suicide and ageing: I. Patterns of psychiatric diagnosis. *Int. Psychogeriatr.* **7**, 149–164.
2. Fiebel, J.H. and Springer, C.J. (1982) Depression and failure to resume social activities after stroke. *Arch. Phys. Med. Rehab.* **63**, 276–278.
3. Silverstone, P.H. (1990) Depression increases mortality and morbidity in acute life-threatening medical illness. *J. Psychosom. Res.* **34**, 651–657.
4. Copeland, J.R.M., Davidson, I.A., Dewey, M.E., *et al.* (1992) Alzheimer's disease, other dementias, depression and pseudodementia: prevalence, incidence and three-year outcome in Liverpool. *Br. J. Psychiatry* **161**, 230–239.
5. Blazer, D. (1980) The diagnosis of depression in the elderly. *J. Am. Geriat. Soc.* **28**, 52–58.
6. Bayer, A.J. and Pathy, M.S. (1989) Identification of depression in geriatric medical patients. In: Ghose, K. (Ed.) *Antidepressants for elderly people*, pp. 13–25. London: Chapman and Hall.
7. Georgotas, A., McCue, R.E. and Cooper, T.B. (1989) A placebo controlled comparison of nortriptyline and phenelzine in maintenance therapy of elderly depressed patients. *Arch. Gen. Psychiatry* **46**, 783–786.
8. Braithwaite, R.A., Montgomery, S.A., *et al.* (1979) Age, depression and tricyclic antidepressant levels. In: Anonymous *Pharmacokinetics in the elderly*. London: Macmillan.
9. Nelson, J.C., Mazure, C.M. and Jatlow, P.I. (1994) Characteristics of desipramine-refractory depression. *J. Clin. Psychiatry* **55**, 12–19.
10. Cole, M.G. (1990) The prognosis of depression in the elderly. *Can. Med. Assoc. J.* **142**, 633–639.
11. Salzman, C. (1997) Pharmacologic treatment of depression in the elderly. *J. Clin. Psychiat.* **54 (suppl 2)**, 23–28.
12. Montgomery, S.A. (1993) New psychotropic drugs for the acute treatment of depressive episodes. In: Costa Silva, J.A. and Nadelson, C.C. (Eds) *International review of psychiatry*, pp. 139–160. New York: American Psychiatric Press.
13. Montgomery, S.A. (1992) The advantages of paroxetine in different subgroups of depression. *Int. Clin. Psychopharmacol.* **6 (suppl 4)**, 91–100.
14. Nyth, A.L., Gottfries, C.G., Lyby, K., *et al.* (1992) A controlled multicentre clinical study of citalopram and placebo in elderly depressed patients with and without concomitant dementia. *Acta. Psychiatr. Scand.* **86**, 138–145.

15. Nyth, A.L. and Gottfries, C.G. (1990) The clinical efficacy of citalopram in treatment of emotional disturbances in dementia disorders: a Nordic multi-centre study. *Br. J. Psychiatry* **157**, 894–901.
16. Wakelin, J.S. (1986) Fluvoxamine in the treatment of the older depressed patient: double blind placebo controlled data. *Int. Clin. Psychopharmacol.* **1**, 221–230.
17. Rahman, M.K., Akhtar, M.J., Savla, N.C., *et al.* (1991) A double-blind randomised comparison of fluvoxamine with dothiepin in the treatment of depression in elderly patients. *Br. J. Clin. Pract.* **45**, 255–258.
18. Phanjoo, A., Wonnacott, S. and Hodgson, A. (1991) Double blind comparative multi center study of fluvoxamine and mianserin in the treatment of major depressive episode in the elderly. *Acta Psychiatr. Scand.* **83**, 476–479.
19. Tollefson, G.D. and Holman, S.J.L. (1993) Analysis of the Hamilton Depression Rating Scale factors from a double-blind, placebo-controlled trial of fluoxetine in geriatric major depression. *Int. Clin. Psychopharmacol.* **8**, 253–259.
20. Feighner, J.P. and Cohn, J.B. (1985) Double-blind comparative trials of fluoxetine and doxepin in geriatric patients with major depressive disorder. *J. Clin. Psychiat.* **46**, 20–25.
21. Altamura, A.C., Percudani, M., Guercetti, G. and Invernizzi, G. (1989) Efficacy and tolerability of fluoxetine in the elderly: a double blind study versus amitriptyline. *Int. Clin. Psychopharmacol.* **4**, 103–106.
22. Falk, W.E., Rosenbaum, J.E., Otto, M.W., *et al.* (1989) Fluoxetine versus trazodone in depressed geriatric patients. *J. Geriatr. Psychiatr. Neurol.* **2**, 208–214.
23. Dunner, D.L., Cohn, J.B., Walshe, T., *et al.* (1992) Two combined multi centre double blind studies of paroxetine and domipin in geriatric patients with major depression. *J. Clin. Psychiatry* **53**, 57–60.
24. Guillibert, E., Pelicier, Y., Archambault, J.L., *et al.* (1989) A double blind multi centre study of paroxetine v clomipramine in depressed elderly patients. *Acta Psychiatr. Scand.* **80**, 132–134.
25. Hutchinson, D.R., Tong, S., Moon, C.A.L., *et al.* (1991) A double-blind study in general practice to compare the efficacy and tolerability of paroxetine and amitriptyline in depressed elderly patients. *Br. J. Clin. Res.* **2**, 43–57.
26. Dorman, T. (1992) Sleep and paroxetine: a comparison with mianserin in elderly depressed patients. *Int. Clin. Psychopharmacol.* **6**, 53–58.
27. Schone, W. and Ludwig, M. (1993) A double-blind study of paroxetine compared with fluoxetine in geriatric patients with major depression. *J. Clin. Psychopharmacol.* **13 (suppl 2)**, 34–39.
28. Dunbar, G.C. (1995) Paroxetine in the elderly: a comparative meta-analysis against standard antidepressant pharmacotherapy. *Pharmacology* **51**, 127–144.
29. Cohn, C.K., Shrivastava, R., Mendel, S.J., *et al.* (1990) Double blind multicentre comparison of sertraline and amitriptyline in elderly depressed patients. *J. Clin. Psychiatry* **51 (suppl 8)**, 28–33.
30. Benkert, O., Grunder, G., Wetzel, H. and Hackett, D. (1996) A randomized, double-blind comparison of a rapidly escalating dose of venlafaxine and imipramine in inpatients with major depression and melancholia. *J. Psychiat. Res.* **30**, 441–452.
31. Clerc, G.E., Ruimy, P. and Verdeau Pailles, J. (1996) A double-blind comparison of venlafaxine and fluoxetine in patients hospitalized for major depression and melancholia. *Int. Clin. Psychopharmacol.* **9**, 139–143.
32. Wheatley, D., van Moffaert, M., Timmerman, L., *et al.* (1997) Mirtazapine: efficacy and tolerability in comparison with fluoxetine in patients with major depression. *J. Clin. Psychiatry* (in press).
33. Georgotas, A., McCue, R.E., Cooper, T.B., *et al.* (1989) Factors affecting the delay of antidepressant effect in responders to nortriptyline and phenelzine. *Psychiatr. Res.* **28**, 1–9.

34. Jacobi, D.M. and Lunn, M.A. (1993) How long should the elderly take antide-pressants? A double-blind placebo-controlled study of continuation/prophy-laxis therapy. *Br. J. Psychiatry* **162**, 175–182.
35. Johnson, D.A.W. (1981) Depression: treatment compliance in general practice. *Acta. Psychiatr. Scand.* **63 (S290)**, 447–453.
36. Nolan, L. and O'Malley, K. (1992) Adverse effects of antidepressants in the elderly. *Drugs and Aging* **2**, 450–458.
37. Ray, W.A., Griffin, M.R., Shaffner, W., *et al.* (1987) Psychotropic drug use and the risk of hip fracture. *New Eng. J. Med.* **316**, 363–36.
38. Montgomery, S.A., Henry, J., McDonald, G., Dinan, T., Lader, M., Hindmarch, I., Clare, A. and Nutt, D. (1994) Selective serotonin reuptake inhibitors: meta-analysis of discontinuation rates. *Int. Clin. Psychopharmacol.* **9**, 47–53.
39. Montgomery, S.A. and Kasper, S. (1995) Comparison of compliance between serotonin reuptake inhibitors and tricyclic antidepressants: a meta-analysis. *Int. Clin. Psychopharmacol.* **9 (suppl 4)**, 33–40.
40. Montgomery, S.A. (1989) The efficacy of fluoxetine as an antidepressant in the short and long term. *Int. Clin. Psychopharmacol.* **4 (suppl 1)**, 113–119.
41. Guelfi, J.D., White, A.C., Hackett, D. and Guichoux, J.V. (1995) Effectiveness of venlafaxine in hospitalized patients with major depression and melancho-lia. *J. Clin. Psychiatry* **56**, 450–458.
42. Montgomery, S.A. (1995) Safety of mirtazapine: a review. *Int. Clin. Psychopharmacol.* **10 (suppl 4)**, 37–45.
43. Kasper, S. (1995) Clinical efficacy of mirtazapine: review of metanalyses of pooled data. *Int. Clin. Psychopharmacol.* **10 (suppl. 4)**, 25–35.
44. Roose, S.P., Glassman, A.H., Giardina, E.G., *et al.* (1987) Tricyclic antidepres-sants in depressed patients with cardiac conduction disease. *Arch. Gen. Psychology* **44**, 273–275.
45. Fisch, C. (1985) Effect of fluoxetine on the electrocardiogram. *J. Clin. Psychiatry* **46 (suppl 3)**, 42–44.
46. Ellison, J.M., Milofsky, J.E. and Ely, E. (1990) Fluoxetine induced bradycardia and syncope in two patients. *J. Clin. Psychiatry* **51**, 385–386.
47. Buff, D., Brenner, R., Kirtane, S.S. and Gilboa, R. (1991) Dysthymia associated with fluoxetine treatment in an elderly patient with cardiac disease. *J. Psychiatry* **52**, 174–176.
48. Spier, S.A. and Frontera, M.A. (1991) Unexpected deaths in depressed med-ical inpatients treated with floxetine. *J. Clin. Psychiatry* **52**, 377–382.
49. Henry, J.A., Alexander, C.A. and Sener, E.K. (1995) Relative mortality from overdose of antidepressants. *Br. Med. J.* **310**, 221–224.
50. Jenner, P.N. (1992) Paroxetine: an overview of dosage, tolerability, and safety. *Int. Clin. Psychopharmacol.* **6(suppl 4)**, 69–80.
51. Fredericson-Overo, K., Toft, B., Christopherson, L. and Gylding-Sabroe, J.P. (1985) Kinetics of citalopram in elderly patients. *Psychopharmacology* **86**, 253–257.
52. Lemberger, L., Bergstrom, R.F., Wolen, R.L., *et al.* (1985) Fluoxetine: clinical pharmacology and physiologic disposition. *J. Clin. Psychiatry* **46**, 14–19.
53. Murdoch, D. and McTavish, D. (1992) Sertraline: a review of its pharmacody-namic and pharmacokinetic properties, therapeutic potential in depressive illness, and prospective role in the treatment of obsessive-compulsive disor-der. *Drugs* **44**, 604–624.
54. Benfield, P. and Ward, A. (1986) Fluvoxamine: a review of its pharmacody-namic and pharmacokinetic properties, and therapeutic efficacy in depres-sive illness. *Drugs* **32**, 313–334.
55. Baumann, P. (1992) Clinical pharmacokinetics of citalopram and other selective serotonergic reuptake inhibitors. *Int. Clin. Psychopharmacol.* **6 (suppl 5)**, 13–20.

10

Physical disorders and psychiatric illness

Chris Krasucki and Declan McLoughlin

INTRODUCTION

It is the common experience of old age psychiatrists that elderly patients, rather than falling neatly into categories of either physical illness or psychiatric illness, are more likely to have a combination of both. This has important consequences for aetiology, diagnosis and treatment.

From the aetiological point of view, it is of value to know whether a presenting psychiatric condition arises from a particular physical state or whether physical illness is supervening on a psychiatric condition, or indeed whether both are epiphenomena of some common but undisclosed process, such as ageing itself. Furthermore, both International Classification of Diseases (ICD) and Diagnostic and Statistical Manual (DSM) classification systems require psychiatrists, when making a diagnosis, to make a judgement on whether the psychiatric condition is based on any intra- or extracerebral pathological changes, i.e. whether it is organic. Such a judgement can only be made on the basis of knowledge of the effect of physical changes on the mental state and vice versa. Finally, treatment can only be effectively targeted if one has some idea of the relative weight to place on physical and psychiatric symptoms, and therefore how likely one is, in treating one set of symptoms, to ameliorate the other.

Psychopharmacology of Cognitive and Psychiatric Disorders in the Elderly. Edited by David Wheatley and David Smith. Published in 1998 by Chapman and Hall, London. ISBN 0 412 82470 1

This chapter discusses special considerations relating to the epidemiology of physical/psychiatric co-morbidity and reviews the different forms that the relation between physical and psychiatric illness can take, with examples from research with the elderly. Explanatory models for the relation between physical and psychiatric illness, and in particular the role of stress, will be explored. Finally, treatment approaches to co-morbid physical and psychiatric illness will be discussed, with particular reference to the work of the old age liaison psychiatrist.

EPIDEMIOLOGY OF CO-MORBID PHYSICAL/PSYCHIATRIC ILLNESS: SPECIAL CONSIDERATIONS

Studies of co-morbidity between physical and psychiatric illness can be prone to certain methodological problems. Firstly, there is an overlap in the symptomatology of the two types of illness which may result in the confounding of the measurement of one with the measurement of the other. This effect may be greater in the elderly than in the general population because of the increased prevalence of physical symptoms and physical illness. Secondly, co-morbidity studies are to a great extent influenced by the various factors that determine the process by which such patients establish contact with medical agencies. For example, patients with anxiety or depression tend to consult their doctor more frequently and have a lower threshold for reporting physical symptoms when they do consult, making the correlation between depressive and physical morbidity more apparent than real. Thirdly, physical illness may delay recovery from psychiatric disorder, resulting in individuals with both types of illness being overrepresented in samples of consulting patients. Fourthly, the apparent extent of co-morbidity will depend on the setting in which a patient is seen. The increase in psychiatric morbidity as one moves from the community to psychiatric inpatient facilities is well recognised. Such a progression in symptom severity may also occur with respect to physical illness, so one could speculate that, even if there were no causal relation between physical and psychiatric illness, the closer an individual approached hospital inpatient status the more likely there would be co-morbid physical and psychiatric illness simply by chance association. Certainly there is evidence that only a small minority of new cases of mental disorder in the general population are secondary to physical disease in primary care settings.

RELATION BETWEEN PHYSICAL AND PSYCHIATRIC ILLNESS

The relation between physical and psychiatric illness can be broadly categorised as in Table 10.1.

Table 10.1 *Relation between physical and psychiatric illness*

	Criteria
• Physical illness with secondary psychiatric illness	1. All somatic symptoms can be attributed to the physical illness 2. Treatment of the psychiatric illness will not remove the physical symptoms 3. The psychiatric illness would not have occurred without the physical illness
• Physical illness with unrelated psychiatric illness	No aetiological link exists between the two: treatment of one would not affect the other
• Somatised psychiatric illness	1. Consultation is for physical symptoms 2. The patient attributes all problems to a physical illness, or thinks that the symptoms constitute the problem 3. A psychiatric illness is present 4. Treatment of the psychiatric illness would alleviate/remove the physical symptoms (All 4 must be satisfied)
• Entirely psychiatric illness	Either no somatic symptoms are present, or the patient considers the somatic symptoms to be part of a psychiatric illness

Adapted from Wittchen and Essau [1]

Physical illness with secondary psychiatric illness

Psychiatric symptoms as a direct consequence of the physical disease process

There are many physical conditions in which psychiatric symptoms are a recognised complication and several psychiatric conditions with established physical antecedents. Neurological and endocrine illnesses seem to be particularly potent causes of mental disturbance. For example, stroke is a common neurological condition, the prevalence of which is known to increase with age. Depression is common after stroke, affecting up to 50% of patients. Research attempting to demonstrate a specific association between lesion site and post-stroke depression has been criticised on methodological grounds. Nevertheless the site-of-lesion viewpoint, in which depression is particularly associated with damage to the left frontal pole, is currently partially upheld. Endocrine conditions such as hyperthyroidism also appear to have a direct effect on mental status. In the majority of elderly people this condition tends to manifest as agitation, and up to half have cognitive impairment.

While clinicians treating elderly people may find that a wide range of illnesses can affect the mental state, there are some conditions that are not always recognised as having a potentially direct role in this. For example, the marked bladder distension associated with acute urinary retention may precipitate acute delirium, which rapidly resolves on bladder decompression. The term 'cystocerebral syndrome' has been coined for this.

It has been known for a considerable time that elderly people with poor vision are prone to visual hallucinations. Charles Bonnet is credited with first describing in 1760 the syndrome that bears his name. Essentially this refers to the phenomenon of formed and complex, persistent or repetitive visual hallucinations; full or partial retention of insight; absence of delusions; and absence of hallucinations in other modalities, all in association with bilaterally impaired vision [2]. The content of the hallucinations may take a variety of forms, be both familiar and unfamiliar, and in most people is different each time they occur. The hallucinations often blend in well with surroundings, but may appear to float in the air or be projected on to a wall or ceiling. Most hallucinate only with the eyes open and sometimes the hallucinations move with the eyes. Patients are often reluctant to share their extraordinary experiences with others, fearing that they may be thought insane and most do not mention them to their doctor. Prevalence has been estimated to be 11% in the visually impaired and there are positive associations with the degree of visual impairment and increasing age. It is this, and the fact that, in contrast to many psychiatric conditions, demographic and social circumstances are less important [2], that has lent credence to a direct relationship between visual impairment and the hallucinations. However, the status of the syndrome has been challenged by recent research demonstrating that elderly patients with Charles Bonnet syndrome may have abnormalities on formal psychometric testing, and neuroimaging abnormalities indicative of an underlying dementia [3].

A similar phenomenon may occur in progressive unilateral or bilateral sensorineural deafness in the elderly. The patient may experience highly organised, vivid and intricate musical hallucinations consisting of a voice or voices, or an instrument, band or orchestra, which almost always reflect past musical memories. The hallucinations are experienced in the deaf or deafer ear, are often of acute onset at a time of further decrement in hearing and are intensified by mental inactivity and low ambient noise levels. In some cases, the tune itself or its speed or volume can be altered.

Such end-organ impairment is also found in late paraphrenia, where sensory impairment has been recognised as one of its most consistent risk factors. Major ocular pathology occurs in 55% of paraphrenic patients and is overrepresented compared with depressed controls, as is hearing impairment. A causative relation is supported by the finding that significant symptomatic improvement may occur in some patients after the fitting of a hearing aid.

Perhaps delirium is the condition par excellence that manifests as a consequence of physical disturbance. The most common aetiologies appear to be stroke, infections and metabolic disorders, a direct relation being again suggested by delirium resolving with treatment of the underlying cause. Underlying pre-existing brain disease seems to be important, and may be found in the majority, and space-occupying lesions, such as tumours or subdural haematomas, occur in 11% [4]. The importance of physical factors is further highlighted by a prospective study of elderly people in which the use of physical restraint, malnutrition, the addition of more than three medications, the use of a bladder catheter, and any iatrogenic event were all independently and cumulatively associated with the subsequent development of delirium [5]. In a similar vein, there exists an important minority of dementias which betray their physical causation by being reversible, or at least treatable. A review of research in this field found that the most common treatable dementias appear to be those related to hydrocephalus, alcohol abuse and brain tumour, whilst the most common reversible dementias are those associated with drug toxicity, thyroid disease, calcium disturbance and hyperparathyroidism, and vitamin B12 deficiency [6].

Depressive illnesses directly caused by the medical treatment of physical diseases

The likelihood of depressive illness supervening on the treatment of physical illness is determined by several factors. The first factor is the nature of the treatment. In particular, unpleasant treatments such as major surgery, chemotherapy or radiotherapy are more likely to provoke a depressive reaction. Secondly and related to this is the uncertainty of outcome. The less certain the outcome, such as in cancer treatment, the more likely is an adverse effect on the mental state. Thirdly, depression has been linked with the need for on-going active participation in chronic medical treatment, e.g. dialysis. Finally, many older people are taking multiple medications and the drugs used may themselves cause depression as a side-effect. The drugs most commonly implicated in the elderly are certain antihypertensives such as captopril and nifedipine; analgesics, both narcotic and non-narcotic; cholesterol-lowering agents; corticosteroids; and benzodiazepines.

Multiple physical diseases may be associated with multiple pains and consequently depression

The risk of developing depression increases with the number of different pains and their severity. This effect may be at least partly mediated by functional disability [7].

Patient may be distressed because of the implications of physical symptoms

Symptoms and illnesses that are unpleasant, life-threatening, conspicuous and acute, relapsing or chronic are associated with a particularly high risk of psychiatric problems. For example, psoriasis is often a conspicuous and chronic condition, which has a negative effect on the quality of life in the elderly that is no less than in a younger age group.

Chronic physical disease may lead to marked disability and thus to depression

There is a progressively increasing risk of disability as one ages. Disability implies subnormal activity, in contrast to impairment, which is defined as an objective, quantifiable pathophysiological condition, and handicap, which is taken to mean the extra burden following impairment. The existence of a relation between disability and depression is a robust finding that is very broadly supported by the evidence [8], and has been demonstrated for all age groups. Different illnesses appear to have comparable effects in producing depression when disability is controlled for, and as one might expect, there is a relation between declining physical status and mental health score [9]. Furthermore, the addition of functional disability to a multivariate model including age substantially weakens the association between age and depressive symptoms [10]. There is, however, a tendency for the relation between depression and disability to become less marked as age advances [8].

Are these findings an artefact of the way depression is assessed? Berkman and colleagues [10] found that physical disability in a large community sample was significantly associated with virtually every item on the Center for Epidemiologic Studies Depression Scale, and not just the somatically oriented items. Also, when four somatic Research Diagnostic Criteria depression items were replaced with four non-somatic symptoms, there was no reduction in sensitivity or specificity of the instrument as applied to an elderly sample [11]. Therefore it is unlikely that the association between disability and depression in the elderly can be accounted for by confounding between physical and psychiatric symptom groups.

Physical illness with unrelated psychiatric illness

While it is difficult in many cases to be certain of a relation, it is likely that in a proportion of elderly people physical and psychiatric illness coexist simply by chance or are seen more commonly together because of patterns of referral to specialist services. Such patients may potentially stretch the expertise of the specialist team looking after them. In general medical in-patients, cognitive impairment is by far the most common psychiatric disorder, occurring in about one-third of those over the age of 70 years. In institutionalised individuals over the age of 65 years, Holstein and colleagues [12] established a similar prevalence of 34.3%.

Hypochondriasis, somatised psychiatric illness and psychiatric illness manifesting with physical complications

Hypochondriasis is a syndrome in which the predominant disturbance is an unrealistic interpretation of physical signs or sensations as abnormal, leading to a preoccupation with the fear or belief of having a disease. Thorough physical examination and investigation does not suggest the diagnosis of any physical disease that accounts for the physical signs or symptoms. Unrealistic fears or beliefs of having a disease persist despite medical reassurance and cause impairment in social, occupational or recreational functioning. The hypochondriacal preoccupation is not due to any other psychiatric syndrome. Research in this area has been hampered by methodological difficulties, which include a lack of consensus on the definition and diagnostic criteria for hypochondriasis, failure to distinguish hypochondriasis as a psychiatric disorder from isolated hypochondriacal symptoms or somatisation in general, and confounding factors that may mediate between age and hypochondriasis, such as life stress, depression and medical morbidity [13]. In particular, some conditions to which the elderly are particularly susceptible, such as organic brain syndromes, may be specific causes of hypochondriacal symptoms. It has nevertheless been suggested that hypochondriasis is common in the elderly [14], estimates of its prevalence varying between 3.9% and 33% [13]. Several psychodynamic mechanisms have been proposed as operative in the genesis and perpetuation of hypochondriasis (Table 10.2).

It is certainly possible that some or all of these mechanisms may come into play as an individual ages, and one could argue that the process of ageing may, by its very nature, predispose elderly people to hypochondriasis. Is hypochondriasis therefore overrepresented in the elderly? When consecutive attenders at a general medical clinic were screened

Table 10.2 Psychodynamics of hypochondriasis

Primary gain
- Withdrawal of psychic interest from other persons or objects, with redirection of this interest to one's body and its functioning
- A shift of psychic anxiety from a specific psychic area to the less threatening area of bodily disease
- Use of a physical symptom as a means of self-punishment and atonement for unacceptable, hostile or vengeful feelings toward persons close to the individual
- Use of illness as an explanation for failure to meet personal and social expectations

Secondary gain
- For varying periods of time, the person receives increased attention and sympathy from friends and health care providers

From Busse [14]

for hypochondriacal symptoms and interviewed with the Diagnostic Interview Schedule [13], those with DSM-III hypochondriasis did not differ in their mean age or age distribution. Furthermore, hypochondriacal patients aged 65 years and over did not differ significantly from younger hypochondriacal patients in terms of hypochondriacal attitudes, somatisation, tendency to amplify bodily sensation or global assessment of their overall health, even though their aggregate medical morbidity and levels of disability were greater. Similarly, there was no age difference in the degree of hypochondriacal symptomatology within the group that had not reached case level for hypochondriasis. There was no difference in the degree of depression or anxiety between the elderly and younger groups.

Nevertheless, the concepts of 'masked depression' and 'depressive equivalents', in other words the expression of depression through complaints of bodily malfunction, usually without any apparent depressed mood, suggest that affective disturbance may be a mediating link between age, hypochondriasis and somatisation. Kramer-Ginsburg and colleagues [15] studied hypochondriacal complaints in consecutive elderly individuals admitted to hospital with severe depression. Of these, 60% had hypochondriacal complaints, 12% of the total holding these with delusional intensity. Hypochondriasis was associated with somatic concerns but, as in the previous study, not with either age or independent physical illness ratings. Furthermore, hypochondriasis was related to both somatic and psychic anxiety, but not depressed mood or suicidality. Further evidence for such a link is the finding that anxiety and a tendency to experience unexplained somatic symptoms may share common risk factors. A large prospective study of individuals aged 70 years and over found that being female, living in an institution, having a low level of social support and having low self-esteem all independently increased the risk of developing somatic symptoms [16].

Drug and alcohol problems are more common in the elderly than has previously been acknowledged [17]. Alcohol dependence in particular is a potent cause of physical complications. Although illicit drug use is relatively unusual, abuse of a variety of prescribed and over the counter drugs may cause physical complications and symptoms. For example, withdrawal from benzodiazepines may cause tinnitus, headaches, tremor or seizures. Inappropriate use of laxatives and purgatives can result in life-threatening electrolyte abnormalities and excessive use of non-steroidal analgesics can cause renal damage. It is salutory to note that the most widely used over the counter drug is nicotine in the form of cigarettes, and approximately 15% of people over the age of 65 years are smokers. Smoking can be considered a dangerous addiction in elderly people, predisposing them not just to increased rates of upper respiratory tract and chest infections but also a variety of neoplasms.

There is evidence that liaison psychiatrists are increasingly being asked to assess elderly people who 'refuse to eat'. Weight loss and anorexia occur commonly in the elderly and may have a variety of causes. Although a wide range of illnesses may be implicated, ranging from neoplasms, cardiac failure and drug toxicity to poverty, ill-fitting dentures or bereavement, in 35% of hospitalised elderly people with involuntary weight loss no physical cause is identified [18]. Anorexia may, however, be a particularly important element in the presentation of depression, dementia and alcohol dependence. Elderly people with depression often comment that they do not enjoy the taste of their food and that they are not interested in eating, either alone or with friends. Frank weight loss commonly occurs. In dementia, changes in eating patterns may occur for several reasons. Patients may have persecutory beliefs about foods they are given, memory impairment may prevent them from successfully preparing meals, or the purchase and preparation of food may be too great a task. Vague complaints of anorexia and weight loss may indicate underlying alcohol dependence or problem drinking. Alcohol has been credited with improving appetite and well-being in institutionalised elderly people, but this view has been challenged and it has been suggested that improved socialisation alone may be sufficient and more appropriate to improve appetite.

While in many elderly persons anorexia can be associated with disease processes, there is also evidence that a true anorexia of ageing exists. Attempts have been made to explain this on the basis of the following: a decreased demand for food as activity levels and metabolic rate are diminished; decreased hedonic qualities of food, in that taste, smell and vision are less acute; decreased feeding drive mediated by a decline in activity of neurotransmitters promoting feeding such as the endogenous opioids and a predisposition to zinc deficiency; and increased activity of satiety factors, such as cholecystokinin [18].

Anorexia nervosa is a rare condition in the elderly but should be thought of in the differential diagnosis of extreme weight loss, especially if there are accompanying psychological features and normal baseline investigations. It is characterised by refusal to maintain a minimum body weight, disturbance of body image, morbid fear of fatness and a preoccupation with measuring and regulating food intake. One population-based study established a lifetime prevalence of 1.1 per 100 000 in women over the age of 50 years, but failed to find any cases in men over that age [19]. These data are supported by case reports of the condition in elderly women, where in half the condition arose for the first time in later life, in one as late as 94 years, whilst in the other half it had originally arisen in youth [20]. That either sex can be affected is suggested by a case report of anorexia nervosa in an elderly man, in whom the condition had arisen for the first time in late middle age. Claims that anorexia nervosa in the elderly may represent atypical affective disorder have been refuted [20].

MODELS FOR THE RELATION BETWEEN PHYSICAL AND PSYCHIATRIC ILLNESS

What is the mechanism that underlies the relation between physical and psychiatric illness? Of the explanatory concepts that have emerged, three will be discussed here.

Control

Physical illnesses clearly vary in the degree to which the symptoms are amenable to control by the individual. Studies show that there are detrimental effects on the health of older people when their control of activities is restricted. In contrast, interventions that enhance options for control by nursing home patients promote health [21]. Is the degree to which a physical illness can be controlled an important factor in determining psychological outcome? Felton and Revenson [22] examined the role of illness controllability and type of coping strategy used on psychological adjustment in a cohort of middle-aged and elderly adults. Contrary to expectation, no difference emerged in psychological adjustment between subjects suffering from illnesses offering few opportunities for control (rheumatoid arthritis and cancer) and those more responsive to individual and medical efforts at control (hypertension and diabetes). Furthermore, while information-seeking as a coping strategy had a beneficial effect on adjustment and wish-fulfilling fantasy had an adverse effect, both of these results were independent of illness controllability. Control as a concept has recently been extended by McWilliam and colleagues [23] who carried out a naturalistic study on a sample of people over the age of 65 years discharged from hospital with continuing care needs. They describe how a lack of clarity about goals, aspirations, purpose in life and a generally negative frame of mind in the elderly patients conspired with the biomedical orientation and paternalism of professionals to threaten autonomy and create a disempowering process. They argue that a patient-centred approach, which should include an understanding of the patient's mindset, goals, aspirations and sense of purpose within a larger life context, is essential to enable elderly patients to maintain autonomy despite continued health care requirements.

Coping

Coping refers to behaviour that protects people from being psychologically harmed by problematic social experience, and may exert its effect in three ways: (1) by eliminating or modifying conditions giving rise to problems, (2) by perceptually controlling the meaning of experience in a manner that neutralises its problematic character, and (3) by keeping the emotional consequences of problems within manageable bounds. Coping strategies in people with serious illnesses include denial, selective ignoring, information seeking, taking refuge in activity, avoidance, reminiscence about former good times, learning specific illness-related procedures, blaming others and seeking comfort from others. Coping is invoked in the stress-buffering hypothesis which maintains that particular levels of stress must be experienced together with an absence of coping in order for the negative effects of stress to emerge. However, Felton and colleagues [24], in a study of middle-aged and elderly adults with chronic illness, showed that the stress-buffering hypothesis failed to explain psychological adjustment, and coping had only a modest effect.

Stress

Stress has many definitions but can be considered in terms of three components: individual susceptibility to stress, stressors and the stress response. Stressors interact with individual susceptibility to produce the stress response. Stressors can be social, psychological or physical. Social stressors often come under the broad category of life events, which are unplanned, unforeseen and usually unavoidable traumatic events for which there is often no time to prepare. Psychological stressors are strong emotions which are usually negative and which may be induced by other stressors or arise spontaneously. Physical stressors are often environmental agents which are potentially damaging but which may be avoidable. Physical illness falls within this category and one can argue that chronic illness in particular constitutes a persistent, damaging but unavoidable stressor.

It is now generally accepted that stressful life events and chronic difficulties can trigger the onset of depression in predisposed individuals [25]. Physical illness also is recognised as frequently precipitating and maintaining depression. Furthermore, the relation between depression and physical illness can be described as self-perpetuating and mutually reinforcing, physical illness leading to depression which in turn leads to physical illness. Aneshensel and colleagues [26] performed sequential interviews on a large probability sample drawn from the community and found that illness had a large, contemporaneous effect of increasing depressive symptomatology over previous levels, whilst depression had a smaller, four-month lagged effect of increasing levels of physical illness. This finding is supported by that of Murphy and Brown [27] who studied a sample of women under the age of 65 years drawn from a general practice register who had recently developed physical illness. They found that in those women whose illness had been preceded by severe life events, the association was not directly causal but was mediated by an intervening psychiatric disturbance of an affective kind, all occurring within a six month period. What biological process could explain such a relationship?

Stress exerts its effects principally through the activities of two major systems: the sympathetic division of the autonomic nervous system, which results in the release of catecholamines from the adrenal medulla, and the hypothalamo–pituitary–adrenal axis, in which the release of adrenocorticotrophic hormone from the anterior pituitary triggers the release of corticosteroids from the adrenal cortex. The principal corticosteroid hormones are the glucocorticoids, particularly cortisol; the mineralocorticoids, particularly aldosterone; and the androgens. These lipid-soluble molecules can freely enter the brain and bind to two types of receptor. Type I receptors bind naturally occurring glucocorticoids and mineralocorticoids with high affinity, while type II receptors bind synthetic glucocorticoids (e.g. dexamethasone) with high affinity, as well as naturally occurring glucocorticoids and aldosterone with low affinity [25]. These receptors are intracellular and the complex formed by the binding of a steroid with a receptor is translocated into the cell nucleus, where it binds to DNA and influences the expression of genes.

It has been hypothesised that corticosteroids exert their effect on mood by this action on type II receptors and the subsequent binding of these receptors to DNA within neurones [25]. It has been further argued [28] that the greater role of stressors in a first episode of major affective disorder than in subsequent episodes might be explained by both sensitisation to stressors and episodes of illness being encoded at the level of gene expression. In particular, stressors and the biochemical concomitants of the episodes themselves can induce the proto-oncogene c-fos and related transcription factors, which then could affect the expression of transmitters, receptors and neuropeptides that alter responsivity in a long-lasting fashion. Thus both stressors and episodes may leave residual traces and vulnerabilities to further occurrences of affective illness [28]. The hypothalamo–pituitary–adrenal axis response to stressors is prolonged or disinhibited in the elderly [29], possibly resulting in greater susceptibility to a process of this kind. Furthermore, a theoretical bridge can be made to cognitive impairment in elderly people. Animal experiments have shown that glucocorticoids have a direct catabolic action on the brain, reducing hippocampal dendritic length and branching. In non-human primates, both glucocorticoid excess and social stress induce loss of hippocampal neurones, and elevated glucocorticoid concentrations increase attendant markers of neuronal degeneration, such as tau immunoreactivity. Although there is evidence linking hypercortisolaemia to age-related cognitive decline in humans, the link between glucocorticoids and neuronal death in humans is as yet unproven.

MANAGEMENT OF CO-MORBID PHYSICAL AND PSYCHIATRIC
ILLNESS

Detection

The first stage in the management of co-morbid physical and psychiatric
illness requires both types of illness to be detected. Although physical illness is often readily apparent or otherwise detectable, both general practitioners and hospital doctors have greater difficulty in detecting
psychiatric illness when physical illness is present. There are obvious
clues which may assist in this task, such as overt anxiety or tearfulness,
but often the best way forward is to arrange a further interview in which
there is sufficient time to inquire about depressive cognitions and other
psychiatric symptoms. Routine psychological screening methods can be
valuable, but only if the clinician is willing to ask further questions to
establish the significance of self-report scores and to determine the need
for further intervention.

Investigation and treatment

Where physical investigation is needed it should be planned, explained
and thus integrated into the general psychological care of the patient. It
may be helpful to suggest the possibility that tests may be negative and
introduce early the prospect of a psychological explanation.

Relatively little has been written about the treatment of co-morbid
physical and psychiatric illness in the elderly. While it is acknowledged
that psychotropic medication can play an important role in treatment of
psychiatric illness in medical patients, there is evidence also that it is possible to take advantage of the unique relation between physical and psychiatric symptoms to effect improvement in both; in other words, to use
psychosocial interventions in the medically ill to improve both psychosocial and medical outcomes. For example, a large cohort study of people
aged 70–75 years living in the community found that uncorrected sensory impairments were associated with a significant and independent
impairment of mood, self-sufficiency in instrumental activities of daily
living and social relations whereas this did not occur in the subjects with
sensory impairments who were using sensory aids [30]. Similarly, physical rehabilitation has been shown to improve mood, mood status improving in parallel with the improvement in disability [31].

A role for the old age liaison psychiatrist

Liaison psychiatry can be defined as that area of psychiatry which is concerned with the diagnosis, treatment, study and prevention of psychiatric
morbidity in the physically ill, of somatoform and factitious disorders and

of psychological factors affecting physical conditions. Relatively little is known about the provision of liaison psychiatric services to elderly physically ill patients. Perhaps because of the increased prevalence of physical illness in elderly people, all old age psychiatrists can be said to be liaison psychiatrists. Nevertheless, one can provide arguments for the provision of dedicated old age psychiatry liaison services. Elderly people in hospital present complex management problems resulting from a multidimensional combination of ageing and, not infrequently, cognitive impairment, physical illness and psychiatric symptoms. These may best be approached through a complementary multidisciplinary approach. With pressure on hospital beds increasing, it is in the interest of both patients and health services that psychiatric difficulties are identified and addressed early, thus lessening distress during the admission and preventing unnecessary delays in discharge. Finally, by accumulating experience with this particular group of patients, we may be able to learn valuable lessons about the way physical and psychiatric illness interact and perhaps eventually what processes underlie this interaction.

CONCLUSIONS AND FUTURE DIRECTIONS

There can be little doubt that in the elderly population physical and psychiatric illness often go hand in hand. While the considerable range of possible associations makes it unlikely that a single process underlies this phenomenon, there are emerging plausible models which hold the promise that in the perhaps not-too-distant future a unifying theory or theories may emerge. Old age psychiatrists are likely to find themselves central to such work, both by virtue of their clinical exposure to elderly individuals with such co-morbid illness, whether in a liaison capacity or not, and through their research. More work is required to further delineate the interaction of physical and psychiatric symptoms over a variety of time scales, and to look for biological markers underpinning changes in both. Although specific interventions aimed at common underlying pathophysiological processes may be unlikely to emerge for some time, we should take advantage of the interrelations we have found to develop approaches that offer effective rehabilitation of both the physical and the mental state. Perhaps then we will have achieved a truly holistic approach for our elderly patients.

REFERENCES

1. Wittchen, H.-U. and Essau, C.A. (1990) Assessment of symptoms and disabilities in primary care, in *The Epidemiology of Psychological Disorders in General Medical Settings* (eds N. Sartorius, D. Goldberg, G. de Girolamo, J.A. Costa e Silva, Y. Lecrubier and H.-U. Wittchen), Hogrefe & Huber.

2. Teunisse, R.J., Cruysberg, J.R.M., Verbeek, A. and Zitman, F.G. (1995) The Charles Bonnet syndrome: a large prospective study in The Netherlands: a study of the prevalence of the Charles Bonnet syndrome and associated factors in 500 patients attending the University Department of Ophthalmology at Nijmegen. *British Journal of Psychiatry*, **166**, 254–257.

3. Pliskin, N.H., Noronha, A., Towle, V.L., *et al.* (1993) Visual hallucinations in the elderly are associated with neuropsychologic and ophthalmologic abnormalities. *Neurology*, **43**, A241.

4. Roberts, M.A. and Caird, F.I. (1990) The contribution of computerized tomography to the differential diagnosis of confusion in elderly patients. *Age and Ageing*, **19**, 50–56.

5. Inouye, S.K. and Charpentier, M.P.H. (1996) Precipitating factors for delirium in hospitalized elderly persons: predictive model and interrelationship with baseline vulnerability. *Journal of the American Medical Association*, **275**, 852–857.

6. Katzman, R., Lasker, B. and Bernstein, N. (1988) Advances in the diagnosis of dementia: accuracy of diagnosis and consequences of misdiagnosis of disorders causing dementia, in *Ageing and the Brain* (ed. R.D. Terry), Raven Press, New York.

7. Williamson, G.M. and Schulz, R. (1992) Pain, activity restriction, and symptoms of depression among community-residing adults. *Journal of Gerontology*, **47**, 367–372.

8. Gurland, B.J., Wilder, D.L. and Berkman, C. (1988) Depression and disability in the elderly: reciprocal relations and changes with age. *International Journal of Geriatric Psychiatry*, **3**, 163–179.

9. Cassileth, B.R., Lusk, E.J., Strouse, T.B., *et al.* (1984) Psychosocial status in chronic illness: a comparative analysis of six diagnostic groups. *New England Journal of Medicine*, **311**, 506–511.

10. Berkman, L.F., Berkman, C.S., Kasl, S., *et al.* (1986) Depressive symptoms in relation to physical health and functioning in the elderly. *American Journal of Epidemiology*, **124**, 372–388.

11. Rapp, S.R. and Vrana, S. (1989) Substituting nonsomatic for somatic symptoms in the diagnosis of depression in elderly male medical patients. *American Journal of Psychiatry*, **146**, 1197–1200.

12. Holstein, J., Chatellier, G., Piette, F. and Moulais, R. (1994) Prevalence of associated diseases in different types of dementia among elderly institutionalized patients: analysis of 3447 records. *Journal of the American Geriatrics Society*, **42**, 972–977.

13. Barsky, A.J., Frank, C.B., Cleary, P.D., *et al.* (1991) The relation between hypochondriasis and age. *American Journal of Psychiatry*, **148**, 923–928.

14. Busse, E.W. (1982) Hypochondriasis in the elderly. *American Family Physician*, **25**, 199–202.

15. Kramer-Ginsberg, E., Greenwald, B.S., Aisen, P.S. and Brod-Miller, C. (1989) Hypochondriasis in the elderly depressed. *Journal of the American Geriatrics Society*, **37**, 507–510.

16. Ho, S.C., Donnan, S.P.B., and Sham, A. (1988) Psychosomatic symptoms, social support and self worth among the elderly in Hong Kong. *Journal of Epidemiology and Community Health*, **42**, 377–382.

17. McLoughlin, D. and Farrell, M. (1997) Substance misuse in the elderly, in *Mental Health Care for Elderly People* (eds I.J. Norman and S.J. Redfern), Churchill Livingstone, London.

18. Morley, J.E., Silver, A.J., Miller, D.K. and Rubenstein, L.Z. (1989) The anorexia of the elderly. *Annals of the New York Academy of Sciences*, **575**, 50–59.

19. Lucas, A.R., Beard, C.M., O'Fallon, W.M. and Kurland, L.T. (1991) 50-year trends in the incidence of anorexia nervosa in Rochester, Minn.: a population-based study. *American Journal of Psychiatry*, **148**, 917–922.
20. Cosford, P. and Arnold, E. (1991) Anorexia nervosa in the elderly. *British Journal of Psychiatry*, **159**, 296–297.
21. Rodin, J. (1986) Aging and health: effects of the sense of control. *Science*, **233**, 1271–1276.
22. Felton, B.J. and Revenson, T.A. (1984) Coping with chronic illness: a study of illness controllability and the influence of coping strategies on psychosocial adjustment. *Journal of Consulting and Clinical Psychology*, **52**, 343–353.
23. McWilliam, C.L., Belle Brown, J., et al. (1994) A new perspective on threatened autonomy in elderly persons: the disempowering process. *Social Science and Medicine*, **38**, 327–338.
24. Felton, B.J., Revenson, T.A. and Hinrichsen, G.A. (1984) Stress and coping in the explanation of psychological adjustment among chronically ill adults. *Social Science and Medicine*, **18**, 889–898.
25. Checkley, S. (1992) Neuroendocrine mechanisms and the precipitation of depression by life events. *British Journal of Psychiatry*, **60** (Suppl. 15), 7–17.
26. Aneshensel, C.S., Frerichs, R.R. and Huba, G.J. (1984) Depression and physical illness: a multiwave, nonrecursive causal model. *Journal of Health and Social Behaviour*, **25**, 350–371.
27. Murphy, E. and Brown, G.W. (1980) Life events, psychiatric disturbance and physical illness. *British Journal of Psychiatry*, **136**, 326–338.
28. Post, R.M. (1992) Transduction of psychosocial stress into the neurobiology of recurrent affective disorder. *American Journal of Psychiatry*, **149**, 999–1010.
29. Stokes, P.E., Mourilhe, P.R., Barsdorf, A.I. and Ombid, H. (1996) Is post stress HPA response prolonged (disinhibited) in aged humans? *Biological Psychiatry*, **39**, 554.
30. Appollonio, I., Carabellese, C., Frattola, L. and Trabucchi, M. (1996) Effects of sensory aids on the quality of life and mortality of elderly people: a multivariate analysis. *Age and Ageing*, **25**, 89–96.
31. Barbisoni, P., Bertozzi, B., Franzoni, S., et al. (1996) Mood improvement in elderly women after in-hospital physical rehabilitation. *Archives of Physical Medicine and Rehabilitation*, **77**, 346–349.

11

Sleep impairment

David Wheatley

INTRODUCTION

Sleep disturbance is an inexorable accompaniment of the ageing process as there is a physiological reduction in the quality and quantity of sleep from the fifth or sixth decade onwards. Thus sleep becomes progressively more fragmented, with an increasing frequency of awakenings during the night. In this context, is it justifiable to use psychopharmacology to change the face of nature? In making this decision, the psychological and physical effects of sleep disturbance must be considered and these are profound indeed.

ASPECTS OF SLEEP DISTURBANCE IN THE ELDERLY

There is no worse situation for an aged person, often denied the comfort of a departed loved one, than to retire night after night only to awaken prematurely in the middle of that night when the safety of sleep had been anticipated until morning. As with a child, so at night all things become magnified: the usual sounds of a dwelling adapting to night-time changes assume a heightened significance of evil portent. The fear of intruders is ever-present and it is small wonder that old people often try to sleep with the lights turned on. Then, far from feeling refreshed from their short physiological sleep, they spend the next day worrying about what is going to happen that night, the next night and the nights there-after. Then, if depression supervenes, as well it may, early morning wak-

Psychopharmacology of Cognitive and Psychiatric Disorders in the Elderly. Edited by David Wheatley and David Smith. Published in 1998 by Chapman and Hall, London. ISBN 0 412 82470 1

ing without further sleep becomes an added burden, an epilogue to the night as disturbing as its prologue.

Sleep architecture

The sleep hypnogram, as recorded by the electroencephalogram (EEG) (polysomnography), reveals considerable modifications to the normal sleep pattern as age increases. The sleep stages are: stages 1 and 2 (light sleep), stages 3 and 4 (deep sleep, delta or short-wave sleep) and rapid eye movement (REM) stage. During the course of sleep these stages fluctuate up and down, most of deep or short wave sleep (SWS) being concentrated in the early part of the night and most REM sleep in the early hours of the morning. Of particular importance is SWS (stages 3 and 4) which in the normal young adult occupies some 20% of total sleep time. As aging occurs there is a progressive increase in the amount of light sleep (stages 1 and 2) at the expense of deep sleep (stages 3 and 4) and REM sleep [1]. These changes are more pronounced in men than in women and some elderly men may not show any deep sleep at all, although it may still be present in women of comparable age [2]. The restorative value of sleep is well established [3] and is confined to SWS. Sleep deprivation inevitably leads to impaired physical and mental performance [4]. Reduction in SWS also impairs the immune system [5,6].

The purpose of REM sleep is uncertain, but certainly it is important for health as after REM deprivation subjects may become more agitated and aggressive [7]. On the other hand, sleep stages 1 and 2 are far less necessary to health and have been referred to as optional sleep [8].

Clinical considerations

There are six main aetiological factors involved in the causes of insomnia [9], to some of which the elderly are more susceptible than others.

1. **Physical** causes involve illnesses that keep the patient awake through the symptoms they induce. Examples are pain, cough, pruritus, enuresis, dyspnoea and others. With increasing age the causative ailments are ever more likely to occur.
2. **Physiological** causes are due to artificial disturbance of the normal sleep pattern, as experienced by shift-workers, long-haul air crews and passengers and individuals who are obliged to sleep under conditions of unusual noise or light. The use of stimulants such as tea or coffee just before going to bed may also keep people awake, as may a restless or snoring bed companion. Whilst the former causes are less likely in the elderly, the latter may be even more common.
3. **Psychological** causes may be even more important in the elderly than the young. We all seek relief in sleep from the everyday worries

that beset us, but often this is denied by the inability to erase those worries from the mind. Thus, the effect perpetuates the cause and in the elderly such problems often assume insurmountable proportions due to declining cognitive functions and reduced financial and social circumstances.

4. **Psychiatric** illnesses are all accompanied by sleep impairment of one kind or another and are more common in the elderly than the young [10]. These causes include: depression, anxiety, panic, phobic and compulsive-obsessive disorders and the psychoses.

5. **Iatrogenic** causes are often due to drugs prescribed for physical ailments. Examples are stimulant bronchodilators and adrenergic agents, beta-blockers, specific serotonin re-uptake inhibitors (SSRIs) and diuretics taken too late in the day, through the nocturnal polyuria they may cause.

6. **Idiopathic** is the term designated for those cases where there is no apparent cause for insomnia. Although the individual requirement for sleep is mutable, with wide variations in duration, quality and depth of sleep, there are occasions when individuals are unable to obtain adequate sleep for any apparent reason. In a number of clinical trials undertaken by the Psychopharmacology Research Group, this proportion was fairly constant at about 25% of patients seeking treatment for insomnia [11].

Sleep apnoea

This important cause of sleep impairment is mentioned but is dismissed in the context of this volume. Psychopharmacology has no part to play in its treatment and indeed sedatives of all kinds, including alcohol, simply aggravate the symptoms [12]. Undoubtedly continuous positive airways pressure (CPAP) is the treatment of choice when symptoms are severe enough and is generally well tolerated by the elderly.

IMPLICATIONS FOR PSYCHOPHARMACOLOGICAL TREATMENT

The first aim of treatment must be to correct any of the etiological factors present, *if it is possible so to do*. Thus, when physical ailments are causing sleep-disturbing symptoms, symptomatic remedies may be employed to alleviate these. For example, analgesics for pain, cough suppressants for cough, antihistamines for pruritus and so on. **Physiological** causes should be corrected whenever possible. Thus, a bedtime hot milk drink can be substituted for tea or coffee and it may be possible to make changes in sleeping arrangements to reduce the effects of external stimuli. Counselling and psychotherapy may help stress problems and elderly people are often unaware of official agencies that may be able to assist them.

Primary treatment needs to be employed for **psychiatric** disorders, as for example an appropriate antidepressant drug when this illness is the cause of the sleep problem. So a compound with sedative properties is usually to be preferred in the elderly. Most of the tricyclic antidepressants (TCAs) cause sedation, although lofepramine and tianeptine may not. Of the newer compounds, trazodone and mianserin are highly sedative, particularly the former; however, the new successors to these drugs, nefazodone [13] and mirtazapine [14], are less sedative and so may be more appropriate in the elderly, particularly in view of their lack of cardiotoxicity compared with the TCAs. An interesting development has been the use of a plant extract, hypericum (St John's wort), to treat depression, reported to be effective and virtually devoid of any side-effects [15]. This might make it particularly suitable for use in the elderly.

In a number of cases it is possible to prescribe alternative drugs to those that **iatrogenically** interfere with sleep. There are no such alternatives in the case of **idiopathic** insomnia and many of the foregoing options may often not be feasible. So the decision must be made to prescribe a sleep-inducing drug, a decision which is perhaps easier to make in the case of the elderly in view of the adverse consequences of leaving their insomnia untreated; but which hypnotic to prescribe?

THE RIGHT DRUG FOR THE RIGHT PATIENT

The normal sleep pattern involves a latency period of up to 30 minutes at most before the onset of sleep, occasional short wakings during the night, a final awakening appropriate to the time of rising, and a duration of sleep of some six to eight hours. Furthermore, the quality of sleep should not be disturbed by restlessness or excessive or unpleasant dreams.

Types of insomnia

It is difficult to obtain an objective *clinical* record of the pattern of sleep during the night. Patients can make sleep–awake records (somnograms) by marking a chart at 15 minute intervals from the time of being ready to sleep to the time of final waking [9]. The records automatically stop when the patient falls asleep and are resumed if waking occurs during the night. By this means, four main types of insomnia can be distinguished, although more than one may occur concurrently (Fig. 11.1)

The type of insomnia is relevant to the choice of drug treatment, particularly in relation to the duration of action [16]. The latter is mainly influenced by pharmacokinetic and pharmacodynamic considerations and, as outlined in Chapter 2, these often differ markedly in the elderly.

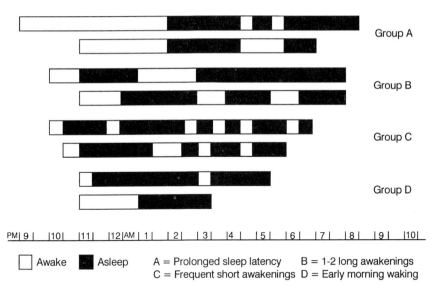

Fig. 11.1 Representative somnograms illustrating the various types of insomnia. Two examples in each group are given. Reproduced with permission from David Wheatley in *Drug Safety* 7: 106–15; published by Adis International, 1992.

Clinical considerations

From a clinical point of view, hypnotic drugs can be divided into three groups according to their average durations of action: *short* (2–4 hours), *medium* (5–8 hours) and *long* (9 hours and longer).

1. **Short-acting** compounds are particularly useful for prolonged latency unaccompanied by subsequent wakings during the night. Thus, the patient is enabled to get off to sleep quickly, with a rapid decline in pharmacological effect so that the natural sleep mechanisms then take over.
2. When wakings do occur during the night, whether these be long or short, few or frequent, **medium-acting** drugs are the most generally useful, combining as they do optimal duration of action with minimal residual effects.
3. When early morning awakening is a prominent feature of the insomnia or a longer duration of action is desirable, then **long-acting** drugs may prove more effective. The usefulness of **long-acting** drugs is limited indeed, although sometimes daytime tranquillisation can prove beneficial in an aggressive or agitated elderly person. There is considerable individual variation in response to hypnotics and there are occasions when the choice may have to be determined by 'trial and error'.

The mean somnograms from a number of clinical trials undertaken by the Psychopharmacology Research Group illustrate this concept (Fig. 11.2). The tracings are shown for a number of contemporary drugs together with their elimination half-lives, an important measure of duration of drug action (Chapter 2).

When choosing a sleep-inducing drug for geriatric use, the *disadvantages* of hypnotic drugs must be carefully considered. These are adverse effects generally and the effects on waking specifically ('hangover'), rebound phenomena, habituation (loss of therapeutic effect), memory impairment and dependence potential. Those who are old tend to be more susceptible to daytime after-effects, to which they are often less tolerant. These will be considered in more detail later in this chapter but generally the shorter-acting drugs are those of most practical use for the elderly.

HYPNOTIC DRUGS

For many decades the benzodiazepines have provided the mainstay of hypnotic drug treatment for young and old alike. In view of current restraints on their use coupled with litigation fears, they are only considered here in overview in deference to the more up-to-date 'non-benzodiazepines'.

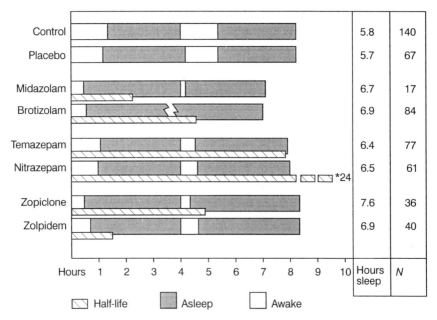

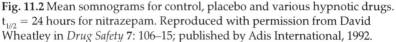

Fig. 11.2 Mean somnograms for control, placebo and various hypnotic drugs. $t_{1/2}$ = 24 hours for nitrazepam. Reproduced with permission from David Wheatley in *Drug Safety* 7: 106–15; published by Adis International, 1992.

Benzodiazepines

The most widely used **short-acting** benzodiazepine is **triazolam** (*Halcion*), which in the UK is restricted to a maximum single dose of 0.25 mg, since the reporting of panic or psychotic episodes following use of higher doses. **Midazolam**, the example shown in Fig. 11.1, has very similar properties but is only marketed for intravenous use in anaesthesia in the UK (*Hypnovel*) although available as an oral hypnotic in Europe (*Dormicum*) and the USA (*Versed*). In addition to the usual side-effects of the benzodiazepines generally, recent memory impairment has been reported with these ultrashort-acting compounds.

Of the **medium-acting** compounds, **temazepam** (*Normison*, UK; *Remestan*, *Silenta*, Europe; *Restoril*, USA) has undoubtedly been the drug most widely used, and abused, at least in the UK. Although potential dependence might be viewed by some as being less socially catastrophic in the elderly, if there are safer alternatives then clearly they should be used. Other medium-acting benzodiazepines which probably have similar dependence potential are **loprazolam** and **lormetazepam** (generic).

There is little if any indication for the use of **long-acting** hypnotic drugs in the elderly as daytime tranquillisation, if required, can be achieved by other means. Examples of long-acting drugs include several erstwhile 'household names': **nitrazepam** (*Mogadon*, UK), **flurazepam** (*Dalmane*), **flunitrazepam** (*Rohypnol*) and **diazepam** (*Valium*) which, although an anxiolytic, is nevertheless often used for its sedative effect; hazardous indeed for the elderly in view of its 24 hours or more duration of action. **Quazepam** and **estazolam** (generic, neither marketed in UK) are other examples.

Zopiclone

This was the first of the 'non-benzodiazepine' hypnotics to be introduced for general clinical use in Europe and the UK (*Zimovane*). A cyclopyrrolone, it nevertheless binds to benzodiazepine (omega) receptors in the brain and has a rapid onset of action with a $t_{1/2}$ of five to six hours and no active metabolites. Importantly for the elderly, it does not reduce SWS and may even increase it. Undoubtedly it is virtually free of waking after-effects but rebound insomnia and tolerance may occur and even dependence [17]. Some of the seminal clinical research on zopiclone has been reviewed by the author [18].

Zolpidem

This imidazopyridine drug with a $t_{1/2}$ of some two hours only has a much shorter duration of action than zopiclone, so it might be expected to exhibit some of the drawbacks of ultrashort-acting hypnotics as in the case of triazolam. Nevertheless, it does appear to be free of rebound insomnia [19] and memory impairment [20], although daytime side-effects may occur which are dose-related and so may not prove to be such a problem in old people [21].

Zaleplon

At the time of writing, this pyrazolopyrimidine compound has not yet been marketed, but it is appropriate to consider its properties here. Pharmacokinetically, it has similarities to zolpidem, with an ultrashort $t_{1/2}$ of 60-90 minutes (including an active metabolite), the principal clinical effect being to reduce sleep latency whilst selectively prolonging SWS and reducing REM stages of sleep. It would appear to be relatively devoid of side-effects and rebound insomnia [22,23], but further and more extended studies will be required to determine whether it has any dependence potential.

Melatonin

Produced by the pineal gland at night, melatonin plays a role in the control of the sleep–wake cycle and serum melatonin concentrations decrease with increasing age. In a study on 12 elderly insomniacs, melatonin metabolism was reduced compared with controls, but three weeks' treatment with melatonin had little effect on the patients' sleep patterns [24]. At the time of writing, melatonin is not available in the UK either on prescription or over the counter.

Other drugs

A number of other drugs have been advocated for the treatment of insomnia, as for example **chloral hydrate** and even still **barbiturates**. These include some, such as **antihistamines, neuroleptics** and **anticonvulsants**, with other main indications but having sedative side-effects. It would not appear that any of these are particularly suited to the elderly, but may be considered as reserve medications should all else fail or the main therapeutic indications are present.

THE OPTIMAL CHOICE

There is no such thing as a perfect drug although some such as life-saving antibiotics come close to it. In other cases, as with insomnia, the harm that the untreated illness may cause (and insomnia is an *illness*) must be weighed against any adverse effect of the drug prescribed to control it. Individual decisions will vary in relation to patients and circumstances and will depend on many of the hypnotic drug characteristics that have been discussed. The overriding precept must always be what is 'best for the patient'. In the elderly quality of life must be a major consideration [25].

So in most cases the decision will be made to prescribe a hypnotic drug with characteristics most appropriate to the case. Some of the disadvantages of so doing may be minimised by optimising the drug regimen. Patients should always start with the minimum dose possible, which may even be less than the lowest recommended one. For example, before the introduction of the 2.5 mg tablet of zopiclone, adequate sleep could be achieved in most elderly people with half of a bisected 5 mg tablet. This was not an easy option given the Lilliputian size of that tablet in the first instance, and the inevitable clumsiness of old age!

When side-effects on waking are a problem, it may be possible to take the hypnotic at a time earlier in the evening before bedtime or it may be appropriate to get up later in the morning. Getting out of bed during the night may pose a difficult problem, as usually this is unavoidable, particularly when due to nocturia. This commonly affects men more than women and any residual drowsiness or dizziness could lead to falls and musculoskeletal damage. A hip fracture that fails to unite is a heavy price to pay for a good night's sleep! Although aesthetically unattractive, the use of an old-fashioned chamberpot under the bed may avoid this. Other daytime effects of a similar nature may be ethically more acceptable in sedentary old people. Further impairment of an already failing memory is not and so becomes an important consideration when choosing a hypnotic for the elderly insomniac.

Rebound insomnia, tolerance and dependence may be minimised by resort to interrupted treatment, as for example omitting treatment for two days out of seven on a regular basis. Such a procedure may be more compatible with the long-term use that is usually needed by the elderly.

CONCLUSIONS

Nietzsche's aphorism that 'sleeping is no mean art: for its sake one must stay awake all day' [26] is particularly apposite for the elderly. For them daytime 'cat-naps' so often frustrate the natural nocturnal state. The oft-reiterated advice to the old not to resist daytime sleepiness may not in fact contribute to their best interests, either psychological or physiological, for the essential periods of SWS are seldom achieved during short daytime sleep episodes and are further reduced during the night. The species *man* possesses cerebral sleep receptors but has either never acquired or lost the ability to stimulate these by cognitive command. If we have not been endowed with an endogenous ligand whereby the state of sleep may be induced, then surely it is a measure of our intellectual purpose that our own ingenuity should supply the solution, albeit by resort to chemical means.

190   *Sleep impairment*

REFERENCES

1. Williams, R.L., Karacan, I. and Hursch, C.J. (1974). *Electroencephalography (EEG) of human sleep: Clinical applications*. Wiley, New York.
2. Nicholson, A. and Marks, J. (eds). (1983). *Insomnia: a guide for medical practitioners*. MTP Press, Lancaster, p. 24.
3. Adam, K. (1980). Sleep as a restorative process and a theory to explain why. *Progress in Brain Research*, **53**, 289–305.
4. Pilcher J.J. and Huffcutt, A.I. (1996). Effects of sleep deprivation on performance: a meta-analysis. *Sleep*, **19**, 318–326.
5. Moldofsky, H., Lue, F.A., Eisen, J. *et al*. (1986). The relationship of interleukin 1 and immune functions to sleep in humans. *Psychosomatic Medicine*, **48**, 309–318.
6. Palmblad, J., Petrini, B., Wasserman, J., *et al*. (1979). Lymphocyte and granulocyte reactions during sleep deprivation. *Psychosomatic Medicine*, **41**, 273–278.
7. Agnew, H.W., Webb, W.B. and Williams, R.L. (1967). Comparison of stage 4 and 1-REM sleep deprivation. *Perceptual and Motor Skills*, **24**, 851–858.
8. Horne, J. (1988). *Why we sleep*. Oxford University Press, Oxford, p. 210.
9. Wheatley, D. (1981). Effects of drugs on sleep. In: Wheatley, D. (ed.), *Psychopharmacology of sleep*. Raven Press, New York, pp. 154–155.
10. Swift, C.G. and Shapiro, C.M. (1996). Sleep and sleep problems in elderly people. *British Medical Journal*, **306**, 1468–1471.
11. Wheatley, D. (1988). Zolpidem and placebo: a study in general practice. In: Bartholini, G., *et al*. (eds), *Imidazopyridines in sleep disorders*. Raven Press, New York, pp. 305–316.
12. Stradling, J.R. (1993). *Handbook of sleep-related breathing disorders*. Oxford University Press, Oxford.
13. Rickells, K., Schweizer, E., Clary, C., *et al*. (1994). Nefazodone and imipramine in major depression: a placebo-controlled trial. *British Journal of Psychiatry*, **164**, 802–805.
14. Mullin, J., Lodge, A., Bennie, E., *et al*. (1996). A multicentre, double-blind, amitriptyline-controlled study of mirtazepine in patients with major depression. *Journal of Psychopharmacology*, **10**, 235–240.
15. Wheatley, D. (1997). Amitriptyline-controlled trial of hypericum in mild-moderate depression. *Pharmacopsychiatry*, **30** (suppl), 44–47.
16. Wheatley, D. (1990). The new alternatives. In: Wheatley, D. (ed.), *The anxiolytic jungle*. John Wiley, Chichester, pp. 163–183.
17. Sullivan, G., McBride, A.J. and Clee, W.B. (1995). Zopiclone abuse in South Wales. *Human Psychopharmacology*, **10**, 351–352.
18. Wheatley, D. (1992). Prescribing short-acting hypnosedatives. *Drug Safety*, **7**, 106–115.
19. Silvestri, R., Ferrillo, F., Murri, L., *et al*. (1996). Rebound insomnia after abrupt discontinuation of hypnotic treatment: double-blind randomized comparison of zolpidem versus triazolam. *Human Psychopharmacology*, **11**, 225–233.
20. Jackson, J.L., Louwerens, J.W., Cnossen, F., *et al*. (1992). Testing the effects of the imidazopyridine zolpidem on memory: an ecologically valid approach. *Human Psychopharmacology*, **7**, 325–330.
21. Miczaj, M. (1993). Pharmacological treatment for insomnia. *Drugs*, **45**, 44–55.
22. Allen, D., Curran, H.V. and Lader, M. (1993). The effects of single doses of CL 284,846, lorazepam, and placebo on psychomotor and memory function in normal male volunteers. *European Journal of Clinical Pharmacology*, **45**, 313–320.

23. Beer, B., Ieni, J.R., Wu, W.-H., *et al.* (1994). A placebo-controlled evaluation of single, escalating doses of CL 284,846, a non-benzodiazepine hypnotic. *Journal of Clinical Pharmacology*, **34**, 335–344.

24. Garfinkel, D., Laudon, M. and Zisapel, N. (1995). Improvement of sleep quality in elderly people by controlled-release melatonin. *Lancet*, **346**, 541–544.

25. Goldenberg, F., Hindmarch, I., Joyce, C.R.B., *et al.* (1994). Zopiclone, sleep and health-related quality of life. *Human Psychopharmacology*, **9**, 245–251.

26. Nietzsche, F. (1883). *Thus spake Zarathustra*. Transl. W. Kaufmann.

12

Paranoid psychosis in the elderly

Brice Pitt

INTRODUCTION

Paranoia literally means (according to the *Oxford English Dictionary*) 'beside the mind, (or, more colloquially, 'beside oneself'), i.e. mentally deranged. The term was introduced into medicine by Heinroth [1] but was first used in its current, persecutory sense by Esquirol [2] when he discussed 'monomania intellectuelle'. Griesinger [3] confirmed his view that paranoia is a disturbance of perception, intellect and thinking, manifest in delusions.

PARAPHRENIA

Kraepelin [4] devised the term **paraphrenia** for a state characterised by morbid suspicion and hallucinations and distinguished from **dementia praecox** (later termed **schizophrenia**) by its late onset in life and good preservation of the personality. Since then the concept has been beset by controversy, which continues. There were arguments about whether paraphrenia was an entity and to what extent it was distinguishable from schizophrenia [5–7] and the term fell out of favour until revived by Roth [8].

Roth described a functional psychosis presenting for the first time in late life, prevailing in about 1% of people over 65 years of age and accounting for about 10% of elderly people admitted for the first time to a psychiatric ward. It comprised a well-organised system of paranoid delusions, with or without auditory hallucinations, developing in a well-preserved, cognitively intact person whose emotional response to the 'persecution' was appropriate, i.e. it was not secondary to confusion or

Psychopharmacology of Cognitive and Psychiatric Disorders in the Elderly. Edited by David Wheatley and David Smith. Published in 1998 by Chapman and Hall, London.
ISBN 0 412 82470 1

affective disorder. Despite a rearguard action by Fish [9] the term became established in the UK at least, though not in the USA [10], where it does not appear in the Diagnostic and Statistical Manual (DSM-IV) [11] or its predecessors.

Post [12] observed that paraphrenia designates a specific clinical disorder, in some ways resembling schizophrenia but arising much later in life, distinct from the other mental illnesses of old age and remarkably true to itself. The question of whether such patients are schizophrenic or not is pretty meaningless. According to the Mental Health Enquiry for England and Wales, first admissions for 'schizophrenia, schizo-affective and paranoid psychoses' (all grouped together) are highest at first in young men, then rapidly decline, while in women there is a lesser early peak followed by a plateau. Both sexes show a drop in middle age, then a marked increase in late life, women predominating, till the highest admission rate of all is for women in their 80s [13]. It seems highly unlikely that the early life disorder is the same as the late life (which must be related to ageing) though there are symptoms in common. Naguib *et al.* [14] demonstrated that the A9 human leucocyte antigen (HLA) which had been linked with paranoid schizophrenia was not associated with paraphrenia, which tended instead to be linked to the B37 antigen, and thus appeared to be genetically distinct.

The writer's irreverent though not wholly facetious view of paraphrenia has been as an 'elderly aunt' of schizophrenia, which allows for a genetic link, the characteristically schizophrenic nature of such phenomena as thought-disorder and passivity feelings and the special susceptibility of women.

The International Classification of Diseases (ICD-9) [15] included the diagnoses paraphrenia, late paraphrenia and involutional paranoid states, but ICD-10 [16] excludes them, so the only categories in which such disorders can now find a nosological home are 'schizophrenia' or 'delusional disorder' and for the present paraphrenia cannot be classified as such for academic purposes. This is much to be regretted [17] because to old age psychiatrists the syndrome is one of the most recognisable and distinctive in their practice. Castle and Murray [18] hold the view that early-onset schizophrenia is a neurodevelopmental disorder originating from faulty brain development in foetal or neonatal life; it is implausible that late-onset schizophrenia has such an aetiology. Instead the term covers a number of disorders [19], some with an illness related to the paranoid personality, some to sensory deprivation, some to organic change and some to affective illness.

Other paranoid states

Paranoid is the principal subject of this chapter, but there are other contexts for paranoia in late life.

A state of suspicion in the elderly is not always morbid. Old people may have drastic decisions taken on their behalf, especially if they are frail, ill and not easily able to speak up for themselves. The fear that they may be moved into or out of hospital, from one ward to another or into a residential or nursing home is not necessarily irrational. Old ladies living alone at ground level on a housing estate may well be subject to persecution by noisy, mischievous children, especially during the school holidays. Confidence tricksters find older people easy prey, muggings are all too frequent and carers sometimes steal. Before diagnosing paranoia it is wise to ask the question 'Could this possibly be true?'. Sometimes it could be and is.

The commonest paranoid state of late life is secondary to **dementia**, and typically takes the form of blaming others for taking what the patient has mislaid, e.g. purse, pension-book, etc. Those most often accused are those closest to the patient: the spouse, the caring daughter, the neighbours, the home help. Sexual jealousy and the Capgras syndrome ('You may look like my son, but you're an imposter!') are other manifestations. Paranoia in delirium is sometimes intense and alarming, but transitory and fluctuating according to the degree of clouding of consciousness. Very occasionally paranoia may be induced by anti-Parkinsonian drugs or steroids. Amphetamine abuse is a notorious cause of paranoid states, but must be rare in old age.

Psychotic **depression** usually involves some paranoia of a punitive kind, associated with guilt: 'The police are following me – they know what I've done!', 'You're going to transfer me to a prison, where I'll be tortured and burned alive for my sins!'. These delusions are not always mood consonant: 'All right, I fiddled the social security once or twice, don't see why they should hound me to my grave!'. Mania leads to paranoia when grandiose schemes are thwarted: 'They're jealous of me – they want to hold me back!'. **Paranoid personalities** have 'a chip on their shoulder' and view the world askance. They are cynical, sceptical, litigious and abrasive, and enter old age alone but not lonely. When they become infirm there are no 'nearest and dearest' to care for them and they either suffer neglect or test the professional and voluntary services by their carping demands and ingratitude. As they respond so poorly to what is on offer, they are liable to be referred to psychiatrists as a last resort.

Prevalence and incidence

Pitt [20] reported that in a comprehensive psychogeriatric service, taking all referrals from a population aged 65 years and over in a defined catchment area, 9% were diagnosed at first assessment as having a paranoid state. The great majority were later diagnosed as suffering from paraphrenia. All cases identified in the epidemiological study in Newcastle-upon-Tyne by Kay *et al.* [21] were found in hospital or residential homes; none was among 208 people over 65 years of age at home. In the same year Williamson *et al.* [22] found paranoid states in two women of 200 subjects over 65 years of age at home in Edinburgh, and Parsons [23] four out of 228 in Swansea, UK. The reported prevalence in these and other studies, summarised by Almeida [24], is 0.1–4%, the prevalence in psychiatric institutions (e.g. Blessed and Wilson [25]) is 10% and the incidence 10–26 per 100 000 people aged 65 years and over per year.

Risk factors

Sex

Although the incidence of paraphrenia appears to increase in both sexes throughout the senium, there is a preponderance in women. This might be due to the loss of the antidopaminergic properties of oestradiol [26] and a relative excess of dopamine D2 receptors in older women [27]. It might also signify that paraphrenia is distinct from schizophrenia and that women are particularly susceptible [18].

Genetic

The risk of schizophrenia among the close relatives of paraphrenics is greater than that of the general population but less than that of younger schizophrenics. Kay and Roth [28] found a 3.4% prevalence of schizophrenia (compared with a general risk of 0.9%) among the kin of 99 paraphrenic probands, and a prevalence for paraphrenia of 8% among their siblings. The frequency of the apoliproprotein E4 allele (a marker for dementia) is less than among normal elderly controls [29].

Personality

Although having, as a rule, a good work record, no tendency to social decline and much less previous psychiatric illness than older people with affective illness, paraphrenics have usually been withdrawn, reclusive, with a limited capacity for closeness and a tendency to eccentricity [30, 31].

Marital status

There is an excess of unmarried women among paraphrenics [28]. Kay [32], however, found that over a quarter of his Swedish paraphrenic patients had illegitimate children.

Brain pathology

Compared with age-matched controls, the brains of paraphrenics show a significantly greater ventricular to brain ratio, less than in dementia and comparable with that in late-onset depressives [33, 34]. Howard *et al.* [35], using magnetic resonance imaging and the DSM-IV classification, found that paraphrenics meeting criteria for 'delusional disorder' were much more likely to have enlarged lateral and third ventricles than those with 'schizophrenia'. While there is no obvious cognitive impairment in most paraphrenics, Almeida *et al.* [36] found some subtle impairments on neuro-psychological testing compared with normal controls, and Hymas [37] following up a cohort of paraphrenics after an average of 3.5 years found some cognitive deterioration, but only two of the original 43 subjects were demented.

Sensory deprivation

The idea that some deaf people may feel isolated, ridiculed and 'get the wrong end of the stick' is plausible. Cooper *et al.* [38, 39], after comparing paraphrenic and depressed older people matched for age and sex, concluded that the former were more deaf, for longer. Corbin and Eastwood [40] found a relation between deafness and auditory hallucinations rather than delusions. Thomas [41], however, found that paranoia among the deaf, as against deafness among the paranoid, was not all that common. Cooper and Porter [39] also found that paraphrenic patients had more cataracts (and more far vision problems in the worse eye) than those suffering from depression.

Being in an **alien culture**, especially where the language is foreign, is a form of sensory deprivation, as is illiteracy. The 'foreign environment' of hospital, where old people in particular may feel baffled, apprehensive, uninformed, disempowered, uncomfortable, restrained (e.g. by cot sides or intravenous lines) and perhaps cognitively impaired (by illness or medication), may conduce to paranoia, notably in intensive therapy units.

Physical factors

The physical factors in paranoid reactions include myxoedema [42].

Psychological stress

This precedes paraphrenia less often than it does depression, but may precipitate a paranoid reaction [43]. A quarter of Kay and Roth's [28] cases were related to traumatic events.

Clinical features

The typical paraphrenic is thus an unmarried older woman of a solitary, eccentric disposition but without a past psychiatric history. She is partially deaf, but otherwise physically fit. She may have a sense of grievance, possibly related to a long hidden 'guilty secret' (e.g. illiteracy, an illegitimate child). In recent weeks, months or even years she has come to believe that her neighbours – usually at one particular address, but sometimes a neighbourhood – are hostile. They comment, criticise and make a nuisance of themselves. Auditory hallucinations are common – voices talking about or to her disparagingly, abusing or plotting against her, spying on her in her most private and intimate activities. She often believes that she is bugged by hidden microphones, surveyed with secret telescopes or television cameras and addressed by cleverly disguised loudspeakers. Noxious gases may be blown in through cracks in the walls, powder sprinkled on her food from the ceiling, her water supply contaminated, her electricity stolen. Visual hallucinations are rare, but there may be ideas of reference related to television as well as radio programmes, or lights flashing in the streets may be thought to be sending messages.

Why is all this going on? The answers are often disappointingly banal: 'They're jealous of my nice flat and want to have it for themselves.' There is frequently a machine operating by day – except when people call on the patient – but more especially at night (this sometimes seems a rationalisation of tinnitus): 'They're drug dealers at work, and they want me out of the way'. One prurient old lady believed that the courting couples in parked cars on whom she used to spy at night, prowling the streets with a torch, were getting back at her. Erotic ideas are an occasional variant on the paranoid theme – passivity feelings of being raped from afar. A widow was distressed by a gerbil which haunted her bed and approached her private parts: she never saw it and didn't really know what a gerbil was like, but was nevertheless certain that one was her persecutor. A poignant, altruistic form of paraphrenia concerns a child being ill-used in a dwelling where there is no child.

Paraphrenic delusions are usually very circumscribed – 'It is those people, at that address' – though they may be systematised, involving everyone other than a barely trusted few. Hallucinations are usually confined to the patient's dwelling, but occasionally follow her wherever she goes – or if she moves to another dwelling. Off the subject of the paranoia patients are pretty normal. They converse normally, if warily, and any thought disorder is confined to occasional metonyms and neologisms – private terms for what is going on, like 'badgerism'. They are well aware of what is going on in the world and carry out the normal activities of daily living within the limits set by their delusions.

Unlike some schizophrenics who amiably live a humdrum existence at odds with delusions of being royal or otherwise special, paraphrenics respond appropriately to their delusions. Having no insight they go, preferentially, to the police. They may turn on their supposed persecutors, who then themselves feel persecuted and complain, so to some extent the patient's delusions become realised. They may seek rehousing or go into a state of siege. Rarely they attempt litigation. They will not readily consult a doctor about the problem for, from their point of view, why should they? 'There's nothing wrong with me – it's them!' Sometimes they repel unwanted intruders with abuse, silence, a bucket of water or an axe kept behind the door! Despite feeling isolated and persecuted they tend not to be depressed, but to offer a spirited resistance.

The writer has visited many old people suffering from paraphrenia. This should usually be arranged by a note or over the telephone, but sometimes it is better to arrive early or late in the day unannounced, where the patient otherwise avoids being seen. Some interviews are conducted through windows or the letter-box, which may at least establish that the patient, though uncooperative and hostile, is in robust bodily health! If the visitor is allowed in, many keys have to be turned and bolts undone. Within the dwelling one may note blankets suspended over the walls to keep out poisonous vapours, cassette recorders set up to catch the extraneous sounds (sometimes played back with the hiss of a blank tape!) and be asked to speak low for fear of being overheard.

Diagnosis

Paranoia secondary to confusion is preceded and accompanied by cognitive impairment, e.g. a mini-mental state [44] score of 24 or less out of 30. When depression is primary the mood change precedes the paranoia, there is often a past and perhaps a family history of depressive illness, and the patient appears guilty and miserable (Geriatric Depression Scale, GDS [45], five or more out of 15; Brief Assessment Depression Cards Scale, BASDEC [46] seven or more out of 21). Boisterous overactivity and a previous history suggest mania. Paranoid personalities have long been so, and their paranoia is more consistent with a jaundiced, cynical, misanthropic outlook than a frank delusional system.

TREATMENT

Paranoia always limits compliance with treatment, so it is important to try to obtain the patient's trust by giving an attentive, sympathetic hearing. Difficult though it may be to gain access, it is best to try to see the patient at home; indeed, there is little likelihood that she will come to out-patients for a first consultation, though she might be seen at her GP's surgery. It is best not to argue or to agree with expressed delusions, but to sustain the impression of keeping an open mind. Having heard the story out, one may agree that the experience must be distressing and explore tentatively what may be real and what is manifestly unreal.

If the patient's experiences, though psychotic, are not seriously disruptive it may be best to let her go on living with them without medical intervention. Possibly a number of such people cope quite equably with their strange ideas, perhaps reassured by the local police that they will look into the matter. Improving hearing with an aid is always worth trying, as is arranging attendance at a club, day centre or hospital; however, long-deaf old people often can't or won't get used to deaf aids, and most paraphrenics are too unsociable to mix with others. Rehousing brings only temporary respite, if any; within days, weeks or months the persecutors are back.

Antipsychotics

Where the problem is more serious, however, the answer lies in antipsychotic medication. This is the reason why, before the phenothiazines, paraphrenics stayed in hospital for months leading to years, whereas since chlorpromazine came on the scene in the mid-1950s the vast majority are discharged within weeks. Post [30] found that of 71 paraphrenics treated with oral medication, 20% recovered fully, 42% recovered but without full insight, 31% made social recoveries despite retaining some psychotic ideas and only 8% made no improvement at all.

How is the patient persuaded to take such treatment – and how can new drugs be tested for their efficacy against old ones in controlled double-blind trials requiring the patient's informed consent? (The answer is given by the dearth of such trials!) The best approach to treatment is to suggest that medication will ease distress and help with sleep under these trying circumstances, until they have been looked into. If the patient had a good relationship with her general practitioner before the onset of the psychosis, then a prescription may well be more acceptable from him or her than from a strange specialist. A community psychiatric nurse may help by befriending the patient, winning her confidence and gradually persuade her to try a drug. As Post [30] pointed out, the patient's attitude is ambivalent and if reasonable rapport has been obtained with the prescriber, treatment is accepted even though it is inconsistent with the delusions.

There has recently been controversy about surreptitious administration of liquid haloperidol in a patient's tea [47]. While it is hard to defend this as good practice, in the real world it is occasionally an acceptable emergency expedient when a more forthright approach might aggravate an already fraught situation. There are occasions, more often in paraphrenia than any other psychiatric disorder of later life, when compulsory admission under mental health legislation is warranted for the sake of the patient and others if she is violent, relentlessly hostile and abusive, facing legal proceedings or eviction or in a state of neglect through staying indoors, besieged. It must be said that the process of breaking into an old person's home and removing her to hospital, struggling and shouting, against her will is extremely distasteful and it takes a long time for the patient to be at all reconciled with those who inflicted this enormity on her.

As a rule one starts with oral medication at home if there is a decent chance of compliance. The phenothiazine thioridazine in divided doses of from 30 to 300 mg daily is a drug of first choice because the anticholinergic side-effects (including sedation, dry mouth and hypotension) are relatively mild. It is, however, also relatively weakly antipsychotic. Trifluoperazine, another phenothiazine, 5–45 mg daily in divided dosage or as 2, 10 or 15 mg spansules, is a 'tried and true' remedy which more powerfully reduces delusions and hallucinations but the incidence of extrapyramidal side-effects (stiffness, drooling, tremor, akathisia) is high and may lead to falls. There is also a risk, after weeks, months or years, of tardive orofacial dyskinesia, which is usually irreversible. Thus the malady needs to be severe for such risks to be warranted. Extrapyramidal effects are reduced by procyclidine 5 mg twice or thrice a day, though the extra tablets may challenge compliance. Most other antipsychotics are of comparable efficacy to trifluoperazine but may have fewer side-effects. Haloperidol, a butyrophenone, especially useful if there is psychotic overactivity, is available as tablets, 3–15 mg in divided dosage daily, as a colourless liquid (0.1 mg/drop) or by intramuscular injection; the risk of extrapyramidal effects is no less than that of trifluoperazine.

Pimozide, a diphenylbutylpiperidine with a long half-life, is given in a single daily dose of 2–10 mg. It should not be given to those with a history of heart disease (which limits its usefulness in the elderly) and an ECG should be taken before treatment because it may prolong the QT interval and sudden deaths have been reported. It is fairly free of hypotensive, sedative and, in lower dosage, extrapyramidal effects, and is specially indicated for monosymptomatic psychosis (like the patient troubled by a gerbil, above). Sulpiride, a benzamide selective for D-2 receptors and the D-3 subtype, in a dose of 100–200 mg twice daily, causes only mild Parkinsonism, anticholinergic effects are minimal and tardive dyskinesia is rare [48]. Risperidone is a benzisoxazole, a so-called 'atypical' agent, a powerful 5-HT-2 and D-2 antagonist, which also blocks H-1, NA alpha-1 and -2 but not ACh or D-1 receptors. It is effective in paraphrenia, perhaps more so than the longer established antipsychotics, with a low incidence of extrapyramidal effects, best given in doses of 1–4 mg twice daily. Howard and Levy [49] have shown its efficacy where there are complex visual hallucinations. Olanzepine is a newer 'atypical' agent, of the thienobenzodiazepine class [50], with a high affinity for dopamine and 5-HT receptors. 5–10 mg once daily is said to improve the negative symptoms of schizophrenia (e.g. apathy and indolence – rare in paraphrenia) as well as the positive (delusions and hallucinations) and to be even better tolerated than risperidone, the only frequent (i.e. in more than 10% of takers) side-effects being somnolence and weight gain.

Because of unreliable compliance, many paraphrenics are treated with depot flupenthixol (a thioxanthene) or fluphenazine decanoate (a phenothiazine) by deep intramuscular injection. This treatment is usually started in hospital, with a test dose of flupenthixol 10 mg or fluphenazine 6.25 mg, and thereafter 20 or 25 mg, respectively, every month. Flupenthixol is perhaps more 'activating' than fluphenazine, and preferable for patients who are or have been depressed. Both drugs are liable to cause extrapyramidal symptoms, falls, fractures, weight gain and tardive dyskinesia, and the commonest iatrogenic cause of admissions to a joint geriatric/psychogeriatric admission ward was found to be depot neuroleptics [51].

Usually hallucinations dwindle within weeks of starting drug treatment and delusions lose their urgency, though full insight is rare. 'They've stopped doing it now.'

Precautions

Neuroleptics are powerful drugs, therefore:

- treat only when the disorder is truly troublesome;
- be especially cautious where there is cognitive impairment or physical frailty;
- use oral medication wherever compliance seems likely;
- use the lowest possible effective dose;
- use anti-Parkinsonian drugs for side-effects;
- reduce the dose as soon as possible (or try 'drug holidays');
- maintain close supervision: it is not appropriate to leave a community psychogeriatric nurse to give regular injections without medical consultations at least every six months.

Prognosis

Over an average of three years follow up, Post [30] found that prognosis was closely related to the maintenance of drug therapy. Three-quarters of those making a full recovery stayed well, but it was possible to stop the drugs lastingly in only 16%. Other good prognostic features were:

- immediate response to treatment;
- the development of insight;
- being married;
- being relatively young.

Untreated, paraphrenia runs a chronic, unremitting course till the patient's (not usually premature) death [28].

Treating other paranoid states

The paranoia of delirium and dementia may require the use of neuroleptics, though in as low a dose and for as short a time as possible. There is a danger of compounding confusion by the more anticholinergic drugs, while demented patients, especially those with Lewy body disease [52], easily develop Parkinsonism and tardive dyskinesia. It is more easy to distract cognitively impaired patients than paraphrenics from their paranoid theme by conversation, changing the subject or structured activity. Where possible one will, of course, treat the cause of delirium – including withdrawing, where feasible, potentially paranoiogenic drugs. The paranoia secondary to mood disorder usually responds to the effective treatment of, say depression but where not wholly mood-consonant, may require neuroleptics also – given as for paraphrenia.

Medication has nothing to offer the paranoid personality except, perhaps, to fuel grievance and outrage. As such people cannot be cured, they are best endured or even enjoyed for their prickly cussedness in a world where so many elderly patients are bemused, depressed or passive!

CONCLUSION

Some old people are suspicious with good reason, but morbid suspicion is, after depression, anxiety and confusional states, the commonest presentation of mental disorder in late life, accounting for 10% of referrals to old age psychiatry services. The basis may be confusion, mood disorder or a paranoid personality, but is most often paraphrenia, a primary schizophreniform psychosis. The term arouses controversy as to whether it is an entity or a group of primary psychoses, including late-onset schizophrenia and delusional disorder. Paraphrenia is, however, well characterised by its late onset in life, strongly held systematised and localised delusions, often with accompanying auditory hallucinations, and good personality preservation. The family history of schizophrenia and paraphrenia is less than that of younger schizophrenics but exceeds that of the general population. Paraphrenia predominates in women of a solitary and eccentric nature, who are partly deaf. A previous history of psychiatric illness and precipitation by psychological stress are unusual. Social measures are of small effect, though befriending helps to gain the trust needed to comply with treatment. Neuroleptics are very effective, but compliance and side-effects are a problem. Newer drugs may be more effective with fewer undesirable effects. Compulsory in-patient treatment and depot injections are frequently indicated. Prognosis is closely linked to the maintenance of drug treatment, but whether treated or not, paraphrenia does not reduce life expectancy nor, although associated with some cerebral changes, is it a prelude to dementia.

REFERENCES

1. Heinroth, J.C.A. (1825) *System der Psychisch Gerichtlichen Medicin.* Hartman, Leipzig.
2. Esquirol, E. (1845) *Mental Maladies* (trans. E.K. Hunt). Lee & Blanchard, Philadelphia.
3. Griesinger, W. (1867) *Mental Pathology and Therapeutics* (trans. C.I. Robertson, L. Rutherford). New Sydenham Society, London.
4. Kraepelin, E. (1919) *Dementia Praecox and Paraphrenia.* Krieger, New York.
5. Kolle, K. (1931) *Die Primare Verruckheit.* Thieme, Leipzig.
6. Mayer-Gross, W. (1932) *Die Schizophrenie.* Springer, Berlin.
7. Bleuler, M. (1943) Die spaet schizophrenen Krankhiltsbilden. *Fortsch. Neurol. Psychiatrie* **15,** 259.
8. Roth, M. (1955) The natural history of mental disorder in old age. *J. Mental Sci.* **101,** 280–301.
9. Fish, F. (1960) Senile schizophrenia. *J. Mental Sci.* **106,** 938.
10. Bridge, T.P., Wyatt, R.O. (1980) Paraphrenia: paranoid states of late life. II: American research. *J. Am. Geriat. Soc.* **28,** 201.
11. American Psychiatric Association. (1994) *Diagnostic and Statistical Manual of Mental Disorders,* fourth edn (DSM-IV). APA, Washington.
12. Post, F. (1978) The functional psychoses. In: *Studies in Geriatric Psychiatry,* ed. A.D. Isaacs, F. Post. Wiley, Chichester.
13. Department of Health and Social Security. (1985) *Inpatient Statistics from the Mental Health Enquiry.* HMSO, London.
14. Naguib, M., McGuffin, P., Levy, R., *et al.* (1987) Genetic markers in late paraphrenia: a study of HLA antigens. *Br. J. Psychiatry* **150,** 124–7.
15. World Health Organization. (1978) *Mental Disorders: Glossary and Guide to their Classification in accordance with the Ninth Revision of the International Classification of Diseases (ICD-9).* WHO, Geneva
16. World Health Organization. (1992) *The ICD-10 Classification of Mental and Behavioral Disorders: Clinical Descriptions and Diagnostic Guidelines.* WHO, Geneva.
17. Howard, R., Levy, R. (1986) R. Levy Paranoid states of late life. *Int. J. Geriatr. Psychiatry* **11,** 355–61.
18. Castle, D.J., Murray, R.M. (1994) Schizophrenic disorders and mood-incongruent paranoid states: aetiology and genetics. In: *Principles and Practice of Geriatric Psychiatry,* ed. J.R.M. Copeland, M.T. Abou-Saleh, D. Blazer. Wiley, Chichester.
19. Holden, N.I. (1987) Late paraphrenia or the paraphrenias? A descriptive study with a 10-year follow-up. *Br. J. Psychiatry* **150,** 635–9.
20. Pitt, B. (1982) *Psychogeriatrics,* 2nd edn. Churchill Livingstone, Edinburgh.
21. Kay, D.W.K., Beamish, P., Roth, M. (1964) Old age mental disorders in Newcastle upon Tyne. I. Prevalence. *Br. J. Psychiatry* **110,** 146–58.
22. Williamson, J., Stokoe, I., Gray, S. *et al.* (1964) Old people at home: their unreported needs. *Lancet* **i,** 1117–20.
23. Parsons, P. (1965) Mental health of Swansea's old folk. *Br. J. Prevent. Social Med.* **19,** 43–8.
24. Almeida, O. (1997) The paranoid states of late life (late paraphrenia). In: *Psychiatry for the Elderly* (College Seminar Series), ed. R. Butler, B. Pitt. Gaskell, London.
25. Blessed, G., Wilson, D. (1982) The contemporary natural history of psychiatric disorder in old age. *Br. J. Psychiatry* **141,** 59–67.

26. Raymond, V., Beaulieu, M., Labrie, F. *et al.* (1978) Potent antidopaminergic activity of oestradiol at the pituitary level on prolactin release. *Science* **200**, 1173–5.

27. Wong, D.F., Wagner, H.N., Jr, Dannals R.F. *et al.* (1984) Effects of age on dopamine and serotonin receptors measured by positive tomography in the living brain. *Science* **226**, 1393–6.

28. Kay, D.W.K., Roth, M. (1961) Environmental and hereditary factors in the schizophrenias of late life ('late paraphrenia') and their bearing on the general problem of causation in schizophrenia. *J. Mental Sci.* **107**, 649–86.

29. Howard, R., Dennehey, J., Lovestone, S. *et al.* (1995) Apolipoprotein E4 genotype and late paraphrenia. *Int. J. Geriatr. Psychiatry* **10**, 147–50.

30. Post, F., (1966) *Persistent Persecutory States of the Elderly.* Pergamon, Oxford.

31. Kay, D.W.K., Garside, R.F., Roth, M. (1976) The differentiation of paranoid from affective psychoses by patient's premorbid characteristics. *Br. J. Psychiatry* **129**, 207–15.

32. Kay, D.W.K. (1963) Late paraphrenia and its bearing on the aetiology of schizophrenia. *Acta Psychiatr. Scand.* **39**, 159–65.

33. Rabins, P., Pearlson, G., Jayaram, G. *et al.* (1987) Increased ventricle-to-brain ratio in late-onset schizophrenia. *Am. J. Psychiatry* **142**, 557–9.

34. Naguib, M., Levy, R. (1987) Late paraphrenia: neuropsychological impairment and structural brain abnormalities on computed tomography. *Int. J. Geriatr. Psychiatry* **2**, 83–90.

35. Howard, A., Almeida, O., Levy, R. *et al.* (1994) Quantitative magnetic imaging volumetry distinguishes delusional disorder from late-onset schizophrenia. *Br. J. Psychiatry* **165**, 470–80.

36. Almeida, O., Howard, R., Levy, R. *et al.* (1995) Psychotic states arising in late life (late paraphrenia): the role of risk factors. *Br. J. Psychiatry* **166**, 215–28.

37. Hymas, N., Naguib, M., Levy, R. (1989) Late paraphrenia: a follow-up study. *Int. J. Geriatr. Psychiatry* **4**, 23–9.

38. Cooper, A.F., Curry, A.R., Kay, D.W.K. *et al.* (1974) Hearing loss in paranoia and affective psychoses in the elderly. *Lancet* **ii**, 851–84.

39. Cooper, A.F., Porter, R. (1976) Visual acuity and ocular pathology in the paranoid and affective psychoses of late life. *J. Psychosom. Res.* **20**, 107–14.

40. Corbin, S.L., Eastwood, M.R. (1986) Sensory deficits and mental disorders of old age: causal or coincidental associations? *Psychol. Med.* **16**, 251–6.

41. Thomas, A.J. (1981) Acquired deafness and mental health. *Br. J. Med. Psychol.* **54**, 219–27.

42. Asher, R. (1949) Myxoedematous madness. *Br. Med. J.* **ii**, 555–7.

43. Retterstol, N. (1968) Paranoid psychoses. *Br. J. Psychiatry* **114**, 533–42.

44. Folstein, M.F., Folstein, M.E., McHugh, P.R. (1975) 'Mini-mental state': a practical method for grading the cognitive state of patients for the clinician. *J. Psychiatr. Res.* **12**, 189–98.

45. Yesavage, J.A., Brink, T.L., Rose, T.L., Lum, O. (1983) Development and validation of a geriatric depression scale. *J. Psychiatr. Res.* **17**, 37–49.

46. Adshead, F., Day Cody, D., Pitt, B. (1992) BASDEC: a novel screening instrument for depression in elderly medical patients. *Br. Med. J.* **305**, 397.

47. Kellett, J. (1996) A nurse is suspended (an ethical dilemma). *Br. Med. J.* **313**, 1249–51.

48. Cookson, J., Crammer, J., Heine, B. (1993) *The Use of Drugs in Psychiatry*, 4th edn. Gaskell, London.

49. Howard, R., Levy, R. (1994) Charles Bonnet syndrome plus: complex visual hallucinations of Charles Bonnet type in late paraphrenia. *Int. J. Geriatr. Psychiatry* **9**, 399–404.
50. Beasley, C.M. Jr, Tollefson, G., Tran, P. *et al.* (1996) Olanzepine versus placebo and haloperidol: acute phase results of the North American double-blind olanzepine trial. *Neuropsychopharmacology* **14**, 111–24.
51. Pitt, B., Silver, C.P.S. (1980) The combined approach to geriatrics and psychiatry: evaluation of a joint unit in a teaching hospital district. *Age Ageing* **9**, 33–7.
52. McKeith, I. (1975) Lewy body disease. *Curr. Opin. Psychiatry* **8**, 252–7.

13

Disruptive elders

Denis O'Mahony and Davis Coakley

DEFINING THE PROBLEM

In most cases there is little doubt about whether an older person is disruptive. It is one of the most common reasons for families and nursing staff in hospital and nursing home wards requesting the presence of the patient's physician. For less experienced doctors, nursing staff and carers, a disruptive episode is often a daunting event, particularly when the older person is disoriented and aggressive. Despite this, rapid pharmacological intervention is not always the best way of managing the problem, as disruptiveness may sometimes be a way of alerting the attention of those around a patient to such immediate needs as voiding a full bladder or rectum, relief from acute stresses such as pain, hunger, thirst, breathlessness, extremes of environmental temperature, etc. In these circumstances, disruptiveness may be unwelcome, but nevertheless appropriate to the patient's needs, and it is usually remedied once the cause of the acute discomfort has been identified and dealt with. Acute disruptive behaviour may be the first sign of an acute confusional state signifying an underlying acute illness. In these circumstances, a detailed and careful medical evaluation of the patient is indicated, and the behaviour disorder should not be suppressed pharmacologically without concomitant diagnosis and management of the underlying medical problem(s). Disruptiveness may sometimes be iatrogenic, as in drug-induced toxic confusional states or the disinhibiting effect sometimes seen with psychotropic drug therapy. Frail older people may sometimes become noisy

Psychopharmacology of Cognitive and Psychiatric Disorders in the Elderly. Edited by David Wheatley and David Smith. Published in 1998 by Chapman and Hall, London. ISBN 0 412 82470 1

and belligerent when confronted with day-to-day care issues in the continuing care setting, such as being woken from sleep at set times, being moved from bed for assisted dressing, bathing, changing of urinary catheters and having to take medications. In these circumstances, occasional aggressive outbursts may be unavoidable but a deliberate, explanatory approach to the patient helps prevent many disruptive episodes, thereby avoiding the need for drug therapy. Most older people, however, become disruptive in the context of a dementing illness. Not surprisingly, agitated disruptive behaviour is among the most distressing symptoms for both patients and their families.

MAGNITUDE OF THE PROBLEM

Secondary psychiatric symptoms are noted in approximately 30% of patients with Alzheimer's disease (AD) living in the community, and an estimated 50–75% of AD patients will exhibit a persisting disruptive behaviour disorder at some time in their illness [1,2]. Aggressive, agitated behaviour disorder is common in nursing home residents in the USA, one study citing a prevalence of 48% [3]. In a questionnaire survey of carers of demented patients in the community, the most serious problem they faced on a regular basis was 'catastrophic reactions'. These included patients exhibiting physical violence, such as hitting out, resistance to care, outbursts of anger, usually precipitated by task failure, and were noted in 45 of 55 families [4]. In a cross-sectional survey of patients with AD, Reisberg *et al.* [5] detected serious concurrent behavioural symptomatology in 58% of patients, in whom 'agitation' was noted in 48%, day-night disturbance in 42%, physical violence in 36%, verbal outbursts in 24%, tearfulness in 24%, misidentification of home surroundings in 21% and delusions of theft in 48%. Disruptive behavioural problems are a frequent cause of admission to nursing homes. Cohen-Mansfield [6], in a small study of 32 patients admitted to one nursing home, found that dementia was present in 20 (62.5%) and behaviour disorder in 14 (43.8%) prior to admission. Thus, disruptive behaviour disorders are commonly associated with dementia, affecting approximately half of all patients at any one time, presenting a major problem to both carers in the community and institutional staff.

BEHAVIOUR RATING SCALES

Although disruptive behaviours are highly prevalent in the elderly demented patient population in particular, there is marked variability both between patients and within individual patients themselves. The intensity of disruptive episodes may also be highly variable and, although most demented patients at some time manifest behavioural disorders, the frequency of severe agitation/disruptiveness is generally low. Nevertheless, a significant minority of demented older patients will present major difficulties to their carers and in these cases the intensity of the disruptive behaviour usually warrants urgent intervention. The decision to start drug therapy is not as straightforward as might first be thought. Which behaviours and what level of disruptiveness require drug treatment? Should all disruptive episodes be suppressed with drugs? Should drug therapy be prescribed only as needed, or should regular therapy be given and, if so, for how long? How is treatment response to be monitored, and how is one to decide that a particular drug is or is not effective, or whether the dose of a drug should be increased or decreased? A number of useful behaviour rating scales have been devised in an effort to specify the particular presenting disruptive behaviour(s) and to quantify the problem(s), so that rational decisions may be made about starting drug therapy and deciding objectively whether a particular drug intervention is successful or not.

The Sandoz Clinical Assessment Geriatric Scale (SCAG) and the Brief Psychiatric Rating Scale (BPRS) were among the first scales to be used in the 1960s and 1970s. More recently devised and more comprehensive scales include the Behavioural Pathology in Alzheimer's Disease Rating Scale (BEHAVE-AD), the Behaviour Problems Checklist (BPC) and its upgrade, the Revised Memory Behaviour Problems Checklist (RMBPC), the Dementia Behavioural Disturbance Scale (DBD), the Overt Aggression Scale (OAS), the Behavioural and Emotional Activities in Dementia Scale (BEAM-D) and the Agitation Behaviour Mapping Instrument (ABMI) Scale [6]. Behaviour patterns may be studied by even more sophisticated techniques, for example videotape recording or actigraph and personal activity monitoring devices may be used to study psychomotor disturbances such as wandering and pacing. Most behaviour rating scales are well validated, but generally lend themselves to research studies. For day-to-day clinical use, the Overt Aggression Scale (OAS) has much to commend it, with its simple division of aggressive behaviours into four categories of verbal aggression, physical aggression against objects, physical aggression against self and physical aggression against others, which are rated on four levels of severity [7]. For more specialised psychiatric continuing care units, the BEAM-D may be more appropriate [8], with its more comprehensive, yet succinct layout with target behaviours (nine in total) and inferred emotional states (seven in total) being rated on 5-point subscales.

NON-DRUG THERAPIES

Disruptive behaviours should not be considered directly equivalent because drug therapy may be more appropriate for some behaviours (e.g.

physically violent behaviour) and environmental adaptation may be more suitable for others (e.g. wandering). Similarly, drug therapy should not be the reflex response from medical and nursing staff when they encounter a disturbed, disruptive patient. Such an approach often obscures the precipitating cause, which may be a simple and easily remediable problem, such as a patient with nocturia unable to find his way to and from a lavatory because of dim lighting, which led to agitation and disruption of a ward where other patients are sleeping. In this example, a bedside commode at night-time or better lighting and clearer signposting of the lavatory may resolve the problem.

Non-drug therapies for disruptive behaviour in older patients may be helpful in the longer term. Wandering, a common behavioural problem for carers of dementia sufferers both at home and in continuing care facilities, may be successfully managed using environmental strategies, such as structured activities throughout the day, an open, safe, series of well-signed walkways clearly marked with floor lines where patients have 'room to wander safely', and locked exit doors where appropriate. Regular episodes of screaming, which were noted in approximately half of all cases of Alzheimer's disease in one study of elderly nursing home residents, were significantly reduced by means of music therapy [9]. Intensive recreational therapy, incorporating music and reminiscence, is believed to be important in preventing the boredom and frustration that result in a variety of behavioural problems, although research evidence for this is lacking. Music and reminiscence therapy has a sound theoretical basis, as memory for music and distant events remains relatively intact until the advanced stages of Alzheimer's disease. Satlin *et al.* [10] have recently shown that demented patients with 'sundowning' behaviour and sleep disturbances, who were exposed to bright light (2500 lux) for 2 hours each morning, had significantly fewer episodes of disruptive behaviour than patients not exposed to bright light. Properly timed bright light exposure is thought to work by inducing phase shifts of the circadian pacemaker and by enhancing the amplitude of the circadian rhythm, both of which are disordered in Alzheimer's disease. As might be expected, in the long-term care setting, the most reliable way of reducing and containing disruptive behavioural problems in elderly demented patients is to ensure a sufficiently high ratio of well-trained staff to patients. An environment that is appropriately designed to maximise patients' freedom to 'wander safely' and minimise the risks of patient self-harm and disturbance to other patients is another logical approach to behaviour problems and disruptiveness in older patients. Finally, physical restraints should be avoided because their use places older disturbed patients at risk of physical injury and is likely to exacerbate rather than attenuate the behavioural problem.

DRUG THERAPY: BASIC PRINCIPLES

The use of drugs to control and prevent disruptiveness in patients of all ages, and older patients in particular, is still more of an art than a science. There are several reasons for this, including the wide spectrum of disruptive behaviour disorders and their variable intensity, the lack of firm understanding about the neurobiological and neuropharmacological basis for behaviour disorders, imprecise definition of target behaviours and the paucity of high-quality drug studies with a randomised, double-blind, cross-over, placebo-controlled design. The literature abounds with case reports and small, open studies claiming benefit from one drug or another, but there are few reliable clinical data with which to formulate effective treatment strategies. Despite the unsatisfactory state of the present knowledge base, the following principles apply:

1. A precise aetiology of the disruptive behaviour problem must be defined, and remediable causes looked for and treated.
2. The nature and magnitude of the problem must be documented accurately but succinctly by attendant staff.
3. Non-drug interventions should be considered as first-line management; drug therapy should only be resorted to when non-drug measures fail or in extreme circumstances where drug therapy is the only appropriate action.
4. Select a drug which will likely abolish the target symptom(s), with the fewest adverse side-effects to the particular patient.
5. Use the smallest dose of a single drug which results in calming of the patient, so that non-drug measures may be employed more effectively.
6. Once started, make a management plan for the use and withdrawal of the selected drug, titrating dose against intensity of target symptoms and adverse side-effects.
7. Toxicity from tranquilliser therapy is particularly high in the older demented patient, so that dose increases should be made cautiously.

Yudofsky *et al.* [11] recommend using the drug most appropriate to the psychiatric symptoms. For example, in patients whose disruptiveness is associated with definite psychosis, neuroleptics are most appropriate. Similarly, they recommend carbamazepine for disruptive patients with complex partial seizures, lithium for patients with underlying manic or cyclothymic disorders, buspirone for patients with underlying major anxiety, and propranolol for patients with primary organic brain damage syndromes. For the most part, this approach may be logical, but these disorders account for only a minority of disruptive behaviour disorders. Also, there is no consensus about the role of beta-blockers in treating behaviour disorders associated with dementia. Some of these drugs have major limitations in older people, such as risk of metabolic disturbances with lithium and cardiovascular side-effects from the high doses of propranolol needed to produce favourable behavioural effects.

MANAGEMENT OF ACUTE AGGRESSIVE EPISODES

The two drugs most quoted in the literature dealing with pharmacological management of acute aggressive episodes are haloperidol and lorazepam. Both drugs have relatively short plasma half-lives and may be administered by oral, intramuscular and intravenous routes. Lorazepam is the more sedating of the two and it may be used to advantage, for example when an acute disruptive episode occurs at night-time and sleep induction is desirable both for the patient and for others whose sleep is disturbed by the episode. During the daytime, sedation may not be desirable for the patient and benzodiazepine therapy may result in falls and injury. If lorazepam is to be given, the starting dose is 1–2 mg, orally or intramuscularly; the intravenous route is seldom used because of its impracticality in most disturbed, disruptive patients. The dose may be repeated every hour until the patient is calm. Lorazepam should be maintained at a dose not exceeding 2 mg three times daily, preferably orally. After agitation/aggression has been in check for 48 hours, the dose may be slowly tapered at a daily rate of 10% of the maximum total daily dose. Relapse with dose reduction demands re-assessment of the aetiology of the behaviour problem, and consideration of a change to a more specific agent to suppress chronic behavioural disturbance. It is not desirable to medicate disruptive patients beyond approximately six weeks with lorazepam because of risks associated with physical dependency and withdrawal.

Haloperidol has long been the drug of choice among psychiatrists and physicians for the acute treatment of aggressiveness or disruptiveness that presents a risk to the patient or others. Haloperidol is rapid acting, even when given orally; in fact, there is little advantage in giving the drug intramuscularly or intravenously, provided the patient can cooperate with tablets or syrup. The starting dose is 0.5–1 mg, which may be repeated every 20–30 minutes until the patient is calm. The patient should then be started on a regular dose regime of 1–2 mg three times daily (or half this dose if a parenteral route is necessary). Once the patient remains in a state of calm for at least 48 hours, the total daily dose may be tapered by 25% of the maximum daily dose. Re-emergence of the behaviour disturbance on dose reduction or persistence of the problem beyond six weeks should be managed as for lorazepam. Haloperidol has the added advantage of being one of the least cardiotoxic neuroleptic drugs available, and is more suitable in patients with cardiovascular disorders than other neuroleptics with significant anticholinergic and alpha-adrenergic blocking properties.

The side-effects of lorazepam and haloperidol may be considerable. Lorazepam, like other benzodiazepines, may cause over-sedation, disinhibition and paradoxical agitation, worsening of memory and psychomotor function, respiratory depression and withdrawal symptoms when given for more than a few weeks. Haloperidol, like other neuroleptics, may be sedative (although less so than the 'low-potency' neuroleptics), causes Parkinsonism and other extrapyramidal side-effects, such as tardive dyskinesia, dystonia and akathisia, and occasionally precipitates the neuroleptic malignant syndrome. It is not advisable to prescribe anticholinergics to counteract extrapyramidal side-effects from neuroleptics in the older demented patient because the associated sedation will likely cause confusional symptoms to deteriorate, thus compounding the primary behavioural disorder. It is believed that the relatively selective cholinergic neuronal deficit in Alzheimer's disease predisposes these patients to adverse effects with anticholinergics [12].

The PRN use of neuroleptics is contentious. It may be appropriate to give neuroleptics as required at the initial assessment stages of a behavioural disorder or if the behaviour disorder is infrequent. The target behaviours should be specified, rather than neuroleptics being administered for non-specific 'agitation', which may have a wide interpretation. If neuroleptic usage becomes frequent, this should signal the need for a regular neuroleptic prescription; however, the use of additional as necessary doses to supplement regular neuroleptic therapy is not recommended because of the likelihood of the target effect not being reached and adverse side-effects being experienced.

NEUROLEPTIC THERAPY FOR CHRONIC AGGRESSION/DISRUPTIVENESS

Pharmacological management of aggression/disruptiveness may be broadly divided into neuroleptic and non-neuroleptic therapy. Neuroleptics have been used for managing behaviour disorders associated with a variety of psychiatric syndrome since the start of their widespread use in the 1950s. Neuroleptic therapy in older patients should not be undertaken lightly because of the risk of adverse effects such as orthostatic hypotension, anticholinergic syndrome, Parkinsonism and tardive dyskinesia. Extrapyramidal effects are particularly disabling in this patient group and are not always reversible on stopping neuroleptic therapy [13]. There is evidence that neuroleptics are over-used among elderly patients in nursing homes in Britain. Recently McGrath and Jackson [14], in a survey of 909 elderly patients in 28 nursing homes in Glasgow, found that 217 patients (23.9%) were receiving a neuroleptic on a regular basis. The majority of these prescriptions were likely to be inappropriate, as judged by the US Congress OBRA (Omnibus Budget Reconciliation Act, 1987) regulations, which statutorily govern the criteria for use of neuroleptics in older patients in US nursing homes. The OBRA criteria were adopted in response to gross over-usage of tranquillisers in patients in institutional care in the USA. Essentially they stipulate that neuroleptics should only be given to patients for definite psychotic episodes and those with behavioural disorders due to organic brain disorder that present a danger to the patient, other residents or staff. The 88% of patients in the Glasgow study receiving neuroleptics inappropriately by the OBRA criteria were medicated for such problems as mild aggression/agitation, wandering, uncooperativeness and insomnia.

Schneider *et al.* [15] have recently performed a systematic, meta-analytical review of the role of neuroleptic therapy in behaviour disorders associated with dementia. In their review, they identified 17 placebo-controlled studies, of which seven used a double-blind, parallel group design. From their meta-analysis, they found a small, but significant benefit from neuroleptics (59% response rate) versus placebo (41% response rate). They also concluded that no specific neuroleptic was more efficacious than any other agent, thioridazine and haloperidol being the most widely used drugs in the studies reviewed. An earlier systematic review of neuroleptics in dementia by Devenand *et al.* [16] concluded that they are useful in controlling symptoms of suspiciousness, hallucinations, insomnia, agitation, labile emotion and aggressiveness. Once again, they found that no single neuroleptic was superior to any other for controlling symptoms. Thus, the issue of which neuroleptic to use largely depends on the prescriber's preference and experience with a particular drug.

Nevertheless, there are a number of important considerations when selecting neuroleptic therapy for the older disturbed, disruptive patient. The starting dose should probably not exceed one-quarter of the starting antipsychotic dose in young, non-demented adults [17]. The more sedating (i.e. the more anti-cholinergic) effects of low-potency neuroleptics may be useful if the disruptive problem takes the form of 'sundowning', i.e. a behaviour disorder that intensifies with the onset of the hours of darkness. Haloperidol is probably the agent of choice for parenteral use in severely disturbed, uncooperative patients. More recently, risperidone, an 'atypical' neuroleptic, has become available and may be useful in disruptive patients with underlying Parkinsonism, where 'typical' neuroleptics would be relatively contraindicated. Risperidone is a benzisoxazole derivative with combined $5-HT_2$ and dopamine D2 receptor blocking effects; it is the major antagonistic action on $5-HT_2$ receptors that principally distinguishes 'atypical' from 'typical' neuroleptic agents. Although the antipsychotic and extrapyramidal effects of neuroleptics are mediated mainly through dopamine D2 receptors, risperidone in antipsychotic doses is associated with significantly fewer extrapyramidal side-effects, and is not known to cause tardive dyskinesia or leucopenia (the latter restricts the use of the other well-known atypical neuroleptic, clozapine). In chronic schizophrenia, risperidone is as effective in controlling positive psychotic symptoms as haloperidol, but is more effective against negative symptoms [18]. Whether the beneficial effects of risperidone on negative schizophrenic symptoms apply to problems of apathy and psychomotor retardation in older demented patients with behaviour disturbances is not known. The recommended starting dose of risperidone is 0.25–0.5 mg twice daily. This may be increased gradually to a maximum of 1–2 mg twice daily in elderly patients. At higher doses, troublesome side-effects arise, particularly insomnia, headache, extrapyramidal and anticholinergic symptoms and paradoxical agitation. To date, experience with 'atypical' neuroleptics in older patients is limited, and well-designed studies comparing them with 'typical' neuroleptic agents are needed.

Depot neuroleptic therapy may appear to have the advantage of ease of administration in patients who often refuse to take oral medication. It should, in general, be avoided in older demented patients because of poor control of side-effects and difficulty with optimal dose adjustment. In the rare instance of patients with intractable behavioural problems who consistently refuse medication, and where repeated non-drug behaviour-modifying methods have failed, depot therapy may be tried as a 'last resort'. In this situation, an intramuscular test dose of fluphenazine (2.5 mg) or haloperidol (5 mg) may be used to assess efficacy of neuroleptic therapy. Following a positive response, weekly or fortnightly depot injections of neuroleptic may be given, starting with one-quarter of the dose used in younger psychotic patients.

Few studies focus on neuroleptic withdrawal in elderly patients. Barton and Hurst found that replacing chlorpromazine with placebo after seven months' treatment in a group of 50 institutionalised elderly women resulted in only slightly increased disruptiveness and agitation when re-assessed after three weeks [19]. In another study of nine demented males, Raskind *et al.* [20] noted that only one patient needed to recommence neuroleptic therapy six weeks after stopping. These findings suggest that neuroleptics are best given for periods of days to weeks, rather than months to years, and that the need for continuing therapy should be under regular review.

NON-NEUROLEPTIC THERAPY FOR CHRONIC AGGRESSION/DISRUPTIVENESS

Several alternatives to neuroleptics have been studied, including benzodiazepines, buspirone, anticonvulsants, antidepressants, lithium and beta-blockers. These are generally regarded as second-line therapy to neuroleptics, where the latter are contraindicated, poorly tolerated or ineffective. As with neuroleptics, the literature is lacking in high quality, controlled, randomised studies of non-neuroleptics in the management of the chronically disruptive, aggressive older patient. The following sections review the role of the various non-neuroleptic drugs.

Benzodiazepines

Benzodiazepines are superior to placebo in controlled trials; however, neuroleptics are consistently more effective than benzodiazepines in direct comparative studies. Most benzodiazepine studies involve mixed aetiology patient groups, so that it is not always possible to extrapolate conclusions to patients with dementia. Nevertheless, there is broad agreement regarding the following principles. Benzodiazepines with short half-lives and few or no active metabolites, such as oxazepam, lorazepam, alprazolam and triazolam, are more suitable than more traditional benzodiazepines with long half-lives and several active metabolites, such as diazepam, nitrazepam and chlordiazepoxide. Benzodiazepines are generally more sedative than neuroleptics, and therefore are more suitable for late evening or nocturnal agitation/disruptiveness. The starting dose in older patients should be one-third to half of the recommended starting therapeutic dose in younger adults, i.e. oxazepam 10–20 mg, lorazepam 0.5–1.0 mg, triazolam 0.0625–0.125 mg and alprazolam 0.125–0.25 mg. Triazolam has a very short half-life (2–4 hours), produces a high peak plasma level and may occasionally result in acute psychotic reactions with resultant increased agitation. For this reason, triazolam's product licence was recently withdrawn in Britain. Lethargy, increased confusion, paradoxical agitation, disinhibition and physical dependency are potential adverse problems with benzodiazepines and should be looked for. Structured daily activities and avoidance of prolonged daytime 'napping' may remove the need for benzodiazepines in the evening/night-time.

Buspirone

Buspirone is a serotonin-enhancing agent thought to act mainly via 5-HT_{1A} receptors. Evidence favouring the use of buspirone for chronic agitated behaviour disorder in older patients comes from a small number of case reports. At the time of writing, there are no substantial case series or controlled trials of its efficacy in the literature.

Anticonvulsants

Carbamazepine is the most studied anticonvulsant. Valproate has also been used recently. Carbamazepine has been available since 1974 for the treatment of epilepsy and trigeminal neuralgia. It is also used as a mood stabiliser in bipolar affective disorder, schizophrenia and frontal lobe syndromes. In animals, carbamazepine suppresses limbic lobe activity and reduces the firing rate of locus coeruleus neurones, these being the putative mechanisms underlying its reported beneficial effects in behaviour disorders, together with some sedative effects. In two small studies, Patterson and colleagues [21,22] have reported efficacy with carbamazepine in aggressive or violent patients with a variety of organic brain disorders, at doses up to 800 mg/day producing steady-state plasma levels of 8–12 μg/ml within 7–10 days. In another small study, Gleason and Schneider [23] have reported definite improvement in patients with Alzheimer's disease and associated severe behaviour disorder resistant to neuroleptic therapy, using a mean daily dose of 480 mg, with a group mean plasma level of 6.5 μml. In one small but well-designed double-blind, placebo-controlled, cross-over study, describing the effects of carbamazepine in elderly female patients with dementia and related wandering and restlessness (but most not actually aggressive), there was no significant benefit from carbamazepine, but the plasma levels were significantly lower (3.4–3.8 μg/ml) than those reported in the open studies showing improvement. More common side-effects of carbamazepine include sedation and cerebellar dysfunction, diplopia and blurred vision (at higher doses), inappropriate antidiuretic hormone (ADH) secretion with confusion and hyponatraemia, and anticholinergic effects (carbamazepine structurally resembles tricyclic antidepressants). Rarely, it causes idiosyncratic transient mild leucopenia (seldom clinically significant, rapidly reversed on drug withdrawal), generalised erythematous rash, eosinophilia, aplastic crisis and lymphadenopathy.

Sodium valproate has recently been evaluated in a small ($n=10$) open study of elderly patients with dementia, given in doses ranging from 375 to 750 mg/day in divided doses over periods of 1–8 months [24]. Based on global impressions from nursing observations, eight of 10 patients were considered to have responded, with > 50% reduction in episodes. Valproate in these circumstances was associated with minimal side-effects. A larger, placebo-controlled, double-blind study is needed to assess the potential of valproate more thoroughly.

Antidepressants

Among the antidepressants, trazodone and citalopram are the agents thought to have useful effects in behaviourally disturbed, older demented patients. Both exert their pharmacological effects principally by inhibition of serotonin reuptake by neurones. The effects of trazodone are more complex, because it has both serotonin agonist and antagonist effects, as well as alpha-2 adrenoceptor blocking properties promoting noradrenaline release. The neurobiological substrate for deficient serotonergic function in Alzheimer's disease is thought to be the known pathological involvement of the median raphe nuclei. There is also evidence of significantly reduced concentrations of serotonin and its metabolite 5-hydroxyindoleacetic acid in the Alzheimer's disease brain.

Nair *et al.* [25] were the first to describe the benefits of trazodone in a group of older demented patients, reporting reduced agitation and improved mood in eight of 10 patients with doses up to 150 mg daily. Simpson and Foster [26] found significantly less disruptive behaviour among four patients (two with Alzheimer's disease) with 'hostility and combativeness', within two to four weeks of starting trazodone in doses ranging from 200 to 500 mg/day. Pinner and Rich [27] described clinical improvement in three of seven older patients with a variety of organic syndromes, within three to seven weeks of starting trazodone 150–300 mg daily, having failed to respond to behavioural therapy, neuroleptics and antidepressants. There is no published randomised, double-blind, controlled study of trazodone in dementia-related behaviour disorder to support its widespread use in dementia-related disruptive behaviour disorder. Side-effects of trazodone include sedation (therefore, usually given at night-time) and exacerbation of epilepsy. It causes fewer anticholinergic and cardiotoxic side-effects than tricyclic antidepressants.

Citalopram has been reported to show significant benefit in a study of a heterogeneous group of elderly demented patients with cerebrovascular dementia and Alzheimer's disease [28]. This was a well-designed, placebo-controlled, multi-centre, parallel group study involving 98 patients in Scandinavia. Patients with Alzheimer's disease (but not those with cerebrovascular dementia) were reported to have improved mood, less anxiety, less irritability, less emotional blunting and improved calm. Alaproclate, another serotonin reuptake inhibitor, in a well-designed, placebo-controlled study in 40 patients with dementing illness (of an Alzheimer or multi-infarct disease aetiology), was not found to be superior to placebo after four weeks' therapy.

There is no firm evidence that more traditional tricyclic antidepressants are beneficial in controlling disruptiveness in behaviourally disturbed patients, except where the behaviour disorder occurs in the context of a primary depressive illness. The possible role of the selective serotonin reuptake inhibitors (SSRIs) in treating disruptive older patients has not been explored.

Lithium

The evidence for lithium in behaviour disorder in older patients is weak. Lithium may be effective in some patients with organic psychiatric conditions but Schneider and Sobin, reviewing the case report and small series literature dealing with lithium therapy in demented, behaviourally disturbed patients, found evidence of improvement in only four of 22 patients with Alzheimer's disease [29]. The doses used in most reports were less than those considered therapeutic in bipolar affective disorder, but nevertheless, the risk of toxicity is considered particularly high in older demented patients. These factors, together with a lack of controlled studies, mean that lithium cannot be recommended for managing the older demented patient with agitation and disruptiveness.

Beta-blockers

There have been several reports of the use of beta-blockers in patients with disruptive behaviour problems associated with various organic psychiatric conditions. Greendyke and Kantor have studied pindolol in doses up to 100 mg daily in patients with organic brain syndromes of various aetiologies. Although patients did not experience major cardiovascular side-effects, clearcut significant benefit versus placebo could not be shown in this controlled, parallel group study [30]. Several other case reports and small case series suggest that propranolol is beneficial in doses ranging from 60 mg to 520 mg daily. Controlled clinical trials of sufficiently large size and quality have not yet been undertaken and, as with neuroleptics, there is no evidence that any one beta-blocker is superior to another. Thus, evidence to support the regular use of beta-blockers in disruptive older patients is also inconclusive.

There is a great need for well-designed, controlled, parallel-design clinical trials of non-neuroleptic drugs for the management of behaviour disorders in the elderly demented population, in particular trials involving carbamazepine, trazodone and beta-blockers. Despite the current lack of supportive trial data, many clinicians use these agents as alternatives to neuroleptics, when the latter are ineffective, present side-effect problems or are considered undesirable in older demented patients with disruptiveness and/or aggressiveness. On current evidence these agents can only be considered as second-line therapy to neuroleptics for the management of chronic aggression and disruptive behaviour disorder.

SUMMARY

Disruptive behavioural problems are highly prevalent in the demented patient population, placing great strain on families and carers and increasing the likelihood of patients requiring institutional care. The nature of the disruptive behaviour disorder must be documented carefully, the patient must be thoroughly evaluated and specific underlying causes must be sought and treated. First-line management should concentrate on non-drug behaviour modification and/or environmental manipulation most appropriate to the specific situation. Daytime reminiscence and music therapy may be helpful in patients with 'sundowners syndrome'. In severely agitated patients, who present a serious risk of injury to themselves and others, immediate drug therapy with haloperidol is usually needed; lorazepam is a useful, more sedative alternative, which may be more appropriate at night-time. Both drugs may be given parenterally if necessary. For chronic problems that do not respond to non-drug therapies, neuroleptics may be given, but drugs should be selected carefully to minimise the expected side-effects. No single neuroleptic is superior to another in this situation. They should be given for periods of days to weeks, with careful monitoring of efficacy and side-effects, and once the patient has stabilised, a plan should be made for gradual withdrawal of the drug. Older, demented patients are particularly at risk from neuroleptic-induced extrapyramidal adverse effects, which may not be reversible in all cases on stopping the drug. Newer, atypical neuroleptics, like risperidone, may have advantages with fewer extrapyramidal problems, but experience in older patients is still lacking. In some circumstances, mainly in cases of chronic disruptive behaviour disorder where neuroleptic therapy has failed and where drug therapy is still considered necessary, non-neuroleptic drugs such as carbamazepine, trazodone or beta-blockers may be considered. Unlike the neuroleptics, substantive, placebo-controlled studies of the efficacy of these agents are not yet available.

REFERENCES

1. Swearer J., Drachman D., O'Donnell B., et al. Troublesome and disruptive behaviors in dementia. *J Am Geriatr Soc* 1988; **36**, 784–90.
2. Rubin E., Morris J., Berg J. The progression of personality change in senile dementia of the Alzheimer's type. *J Am Geriatr Soc* 1987; **35**, 721–5.
3. Chandler J.D., Chandler J.E. The prevalence of neuropsychiatric disorders in a nursing home population. *J Geriatr Psychiatry Neurol* 1988; **1**, 71–6.
4. Rabins P.V., Mace N.L., Lucas M.J. The impact of dementia on the family. *JAMA* 1982; **248**, 333–5.
5. Reisberg B., Borenstein J., Salob S.P., et al. Behavioral symptoms in Alzheimer's disease: phenomenology and treatment. *J Clin Psychiatry* 1987; **48** (Suppl 5): 9–15.
6. Cohen-Mansfield J. Assessment of disruptive behavior/agitation in the elderly: function, methods, and difficulties. *J Geriatr Psychiatr Neurol* 1995; **8**, 52–60.
7. Yudofsky S.C., Silver J.M., Jackson W., et al. The Overt Aggression Scale: an operationalised rating scale for verbal and physical aggression. *Am J Psychiatry* 1986; **143**, 35–9.
8. Sinha D., Zemlan F.P., Nelson S., et al. A new scale for assessing behavioral agitation in dementia. *Psychiatry Res* 1992; **41**, 73–88.
9. Cohen-Mansfield J., Werner P., Marx M.S. Sceaming in nursing home residents. *J Am Geriatr Soc* 1990; **38**, 785–92.
10. Satlin A., Volicer L., Ross V., et al. Bright light treatment of behavioral and sleep disturbances in patients with Alzheimer's disease. *Am J Psychiatry* 1992; **149**, 1028–32.
11. Yudofsky S.C., Silver J.M., Hales R.E. Pharmacologic management of aggression in the elderly. *J Clin Psychiatry* 1990; **51** (Suppl 10): 22–8.
12. Sunderland T., Tariot P., Cohen R., et al. Anticholinergic sensitivity in patients with dementia of Alzheimer type and age-matched controls. *Arch Gen Psychiatry* 1987; **44**, 418–26.

13. Stephen P.J., Williamson J. Drug-induced parkinsonism in the elderly. *Lancet* 1984; ii: 1082–3.
14. McGrath A.M., Jackson G.A. Survey of neuroleptic prescribing in residents of nursing homes in Glasgow. *Br Med J* 1996; **312**, 611–12.
15. Schneider L.S., Pollock V.E., Lyness S.A. A meta-analysis of controlled trials of neuroleptic treatment of dementia. *J Am Geriatr Soc* 1990; **38**, 553–63.
16. Devenand D.P., Sackeim H.A., Mayeux R. Psychosis., behavioral disturbance and use of neuroleptics in dementia. *Compr Psychiatry* 1988; **29**, 387–401.
17. Carey-Bloom J., Galasko D. Adjunctive therapy in patients with Alzheimer's disease. *Drugs and Aging* 1995; **7**, 79–87.
18. Chouinard G., Jones B., Remington G., *et al*. A Canadian multicenter placebo-controlled study of fixed doses of risperidone and haloperidol in the treatment of chronic schizophrenic patients. *J Clin Psychopharmacol* 1993; **13**, 25–40.
19. Barton R., Hurst L. Unnecessary use of tranquilizers in elderly patients. *Br J Psychiatry* 1966; **112**, 989–90.
20. Raskind M., Risse S., Lampe T. Dementia and antipsychotic drugs. *J Clin Psychiatry 1987; 48* (Suppl); 16–18.
21. Patterson J.F. Carbamazepine for assaultive patients with organic brain disease. *Psychosomatics* 1987; **28**, 579–81.
22. Patterson J.F. A preliminary study of carbamazepine in the treatment of assaultive patients with dementia. *J Geriatr Psychiatr Neurol* 1988; **1**, 21–3.
23. Gleason R., Schneider L.S. Carbamazepine treatment of agitation in Alzheimer's outpatients refractory to neuroleptics. J Clin Psychiatry 1990; **51**, 115–18.
24. Lott A.D., McElroy S.L., Keys M.A. Valproate in the treatment of behavioral agitation in elderly patients with dementia. *J Neuropsychiatr Clin Neurosci* 1995; **7**, 314–19.
25. Nair N.P.V., Ban T.A., Hontela S., Clarke M.A. Trazodone in the treatment of organic brain syndromes with special reference to psychogeriatrics. *Curr Therapeut Res* 1973; **15** (Suppl 1 OS): 769–75.
26. Simpson D.M., Foster D. Improvement in organically disturbed behavior with trazodone treatment. *J Clin Psychiatry* 1986; **47**, 191–3.
27. Pinner E., Rich C. Effects of trazodone on aggressive behavior in seven patients with organic mental disorders. *Am J Psychiatry* 1988; **145**, 1295–6.
28. Nyth A.L., Gottfries C.G. The clinical efficacy of citalopram in treatment of emotional disturbances in dementia disorders. A Nordic multicentre study. *Br J Psychiatry* 1990; **157**, 894–901.
29. Schneider L.S., Sobin P. Non-neuroleptic treatment of behavioural symptoms and agitation in Alzheimer's disease and the other dementias. *Psychopharmacol Bull* 1992; **28**, 71–9.
30. Greendyke R.M., Kantor D.R. Therapeutic effects of pindolol on behavioral disturbances associated with organic brain disease: a double blind study. *J Clin Psychiatry* 1986; **47**, 423–6.

FURTHER READING

1. Leibovici A., Tariot P.N. Agitation associated with dementia: a systematic approach to treatment. *Psychopharmacol Bull* 1988; **24**, 49–53.
2. Schneider L.S., Sobin P.B. Non-neuroleptic medications in the management of agitation in dementia: a selective review. In: *Geriatric Psychiatry: Key Research Topics for Clinicians*, E. Murphy and G. Alexopoulos, eds, Chichester, London, 1995, pp. 127–52.
3. Zaleon C.R., Guthrie SK. Antipsychotic drug use in older patients. *Am J Hosp Pharm* 1994; **51**, 2917–43.

Index